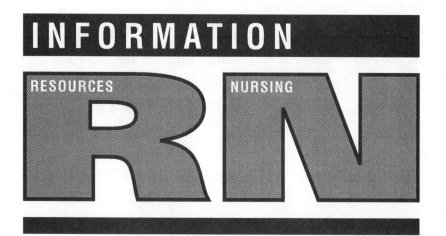

INFORMATION
RESOURCES NURSING
RN

Marilyn P. Verhey
June R. Levy
Russell Schmidt

Cinahl Information Systems
Glendale, California

Information RN

Published in the United States.

ISBN: 0-910478-60-0

Cinahl Information Systems
Glendale Adventist Medical Center
1509 Wilson Terrace
Glendale, CA 91206

1-800-959-7167

Myrna S. Esposo	Production
Elizabeth C. Camiñas	Production Assistant
Peter V. Pravikoff	Proofreader
Ernest R. Razo	Graphic Designer & Cover Design

About the Authors

Marilyn P. Verhey, PhD, RN, CS, is a Professor at the San Francisco State University School of Nursing. She received her baccalaureate in nursing, a master's degree in community mental health nursing and her doctorate in curriculum, instruction, and administration from Boston College. Dr. Verhey also holds a master's degree in library science from the University of Illinois, and has a strong interest in the development of information literacy for lifelong learning in nursing. She has consulted, written, and presented extensively in the areas of patient education, staff development, quality management, and program planning and evaluation, and has practiced as a staff nurse and as a clinical nurse specialist in psychiatric-mental health nursing. She has also worked as a librarian, both in public libraries and at the Biomedical Library at the University of California, Los Angeles. Prior to joining the faculty at San Francisco State University, she was the Associate Administrator for Nursing Education, Quality Assurance, and Research at McLean Hospital in Belmont, MA.

June R. Levy, MLS, is the managing director of Glendale Adventist Medical Center Library and Cinahl Information Systems, Glendale, California. She received her baccalaureate in humanities and a master's degree in library science in South Africa. She has written and presented on searching strategies and the effective retrieval of information. She has worked in public, law, and medical libraries. Prior to joining her current position she worked as a medical librarian at the University of Natal Medical School and as a paralegal at a law firm, both in Durban, South Africa.

Russell Schmidt, MSN, MA, RN, is currently working as an inpatient medical-surgical nurse at St. Francis Memorial Hospital and as an outpatient cardiac rehabilitation nurse at California Pacific Medical Center, both in San Francisco. He has also worked with Dr. Dean Ornish's Preventive Medicine Research Institute in Sausalito, CA as a cardiac rehabilitation specialist, and in the Medical Assistant Training Program at the Mission Language and Vocational School in San Francisco as an instructor. Mr. Schmidt received his Master of Science in Nursing in 1998 from San Francisco State University. Prior to his career in nursing, he earned his MA degree in Systematic Theology from Pacific School of Religion in Berkeley, CA and worked for eight years in the administration of substance abuse programs in San Francisco, CA, Reno, NV, and Providence, RI.

Table of Contents

Introduction

We are practicing nursing in exciting times! The Information Age has influenced nursing and health care information and knowledge in a way we could never have predicted. In just the past decade we have learned to care for patients living with AIDS, conduct our practice in the managed care environment, and incorporate case management in our nursing care delivery systems. These are but three examples of major practice shifts that have required us to learn new interventions, new skills, and new ways of organizing nursing care.

One of the most important skills to be obtained in basic nursing education today is the ability to learn how to locate, evaluate, and use information. Much of what is today's state-of-the-art nursing practice will soon be obsolete, and new concepts, information, and knowledge will be developed. Nurses must know how to obtain new information and transform that information into knowledge over the lifetime of their careers.

The first step toward lifelong learning in nursing is the ability to locate information through searching the literature. This book was written to give nurses and nursing students a hands-on guide to developing skills to access the wonderful, ever-expanding, (and sometimes overwhelming!) literature of nursing and health care. The guide is organized into six chapters. The first chapter is an introduction to locating and evaluating information, Nursing and the Need for Information, the second is Searching the Literature for Information, and the third chapter is Search Formulation: The Six Steps. The fourth chapter presents the Anatomy of a Citation followed by Advanced Concepts for Searching the literature. The sixth chapter presents 24 case studies based on actual nursing practice and developed within a concept and content matrix. These case studies present a hands-on opportunity for users of this guide to practice their searching skills while thinking about "real life" clinical and nursing practice issues.

Information, properly evaluated and used, leads to nursing knowledge, and knowledge brings power to our profession. We hope that this guide will provide a helpful first step in that process.

Nursing and the Need for Information

magine that you are a staff nurse caring for clients from many culturally diverse groups. You believe that your nursing interventions would be more effective if you had information about cultural differences in beliefs about health and illness. You consult your nursing school textbooks, but they do not contain the information you need. You wonder if there are articles in nursing and health care journals that would give you the most recent perspective on nurses' experiences in caring for culturally diverse clients.

You go to the medical center library and use the computer to search for current articles on the nursing care of culturally diverse clients. Within a few minutes you locate several articles on the topic and two of them are just what you had in mind. You copy down the references and make plans to return to read them during your break.

Ponder this quotation…

"In an era when today's truths become tomorrow's outdated concepts, individuals who are unable to gather pertinent information are equally illiterate as those who are unable to read or write."

Gee & Breivik, p.5-6[1]

The preceding scenario is an example of the need for information that you will encounter over and over throughout your nursing career. The information and technology explosion of recent decades requires that nurses engage in lifelong learning to maintain competence in theory and practice. It is important that you know how to:

1 Find information to answer clinical questions that arise as you practice nursing.
2 Keep abreast of the most current research in nursing and other allied health care fields.
3 Continue to learn about clinical and professional issues.

One of the primary ways to meet these three goals is to access resources such as current journals, books, and other materials. This self-study guide will teach you to become an effective and knowledgeable user of nursing information resources. With these skills you will be able to find current information and engage in continuing learning as you practice nursing in an ever-changing health care environment.

As we move into the 21st century, nurses need to know how to find the information they need to remain current and competent as changes occur in health systems, technology, and the delivery of patient care.

SELECTING APPROPRIATE INFORMATION RESOURCES

Many different kinds of resources can give you information about nursing and health care. The resources you select will depend on many factors including your topic, the amount of detail you are seeking, how current you wish the information to be, the use for which you are seeking the information, and the availability of the resource. Various information resources are described in the following section.

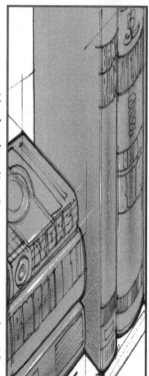

Books
Textbooks

A current textbook is an excellent place to start if you seek an overview of a nursing topic. A textbook is written to be used as a major teaching aid for an academic course. It is a synthesis of the current knowledge and content from established disciplines such as nursing, and is designed to make the content accessible to people unfamiliar with the field. As long as the textbook is up-to-date it can serve as a useful beginning reference tool.

Books

A wide variety of books on nursing and related topics are published every year. Some of these books are on fairly specific subjects (for example, *Fluid and Electrolyte Balance: Nursing Considerations,* by Norma M. Metheny), while others provide an overview of nursing issues (for example, *Nursing in Today's World: Challenges, Issues, Trends* by Janice R. Ellis and Celia L. Hartley).

Reference Books

Reference sources are information tools such as dictionaries, encyclopedias, bibliographies, directories, drug handbooks, statistical compilations, handbooks, and manuals. A reference book is used to answer specific questions, rather than being read cover to cover. The Interagency Council on Library Resources for Nursing publishes a list of "Essential Nursing References" biennially in the journal *N & HC: Perspectives on Community*.

Locating Books

You can find books by consulting the card catalog or online catalog of a library. Ask the librarian if you need assistance. If you wish to purchase a book, consult a bookstore or call the publisher directly. Many publishers have a toll-free number for ordering. Call 1-800-555-1212 for toll-free number directory assistance. If you are not sure whether the book you want is still being published (in print), or if you wish to check on the book's name, author, or publisher, you can also consult a reference called *Books in Print*. It lists all English-language books currently being published or distributed in the United States by author, title, and subject. You can find Books in Print in the reference section of your library, or in most bookstores.

Evaluating Textbooks and Other Books

Two nursing journals publish lists of textbooks and other books that you can use as guides to quality books on nursing topics. *The American Journal of Nursing* (AJN) publishes a list of its "Books of the Year" in every January issue. Since 1979 *Nursing Outlook* has published a list every other year of books (and journals) compiled by Alfred N. Brandon and Dorothy R. Hill. This list is intended to be a guideline for nurses and librarians to use in making choices for purchase. Hill continues to monitor what is being published, and chooses books for the list on a wide variety of nursing topics. Of course, many important and worthwhile books are published that do not appear on either of these lists.

It is important that you evaluate a book to determine if it covers the topic about which you are seeking information in sufficient breadth and depth, and to determine if the coverage is of sufficient quality.

When you are deciding whether the contents of a book are useful to you, there are some steps you can take to make that decision without reading the entire book[2].

1 A preface, foreword, or introduction will often provide a summary of the approach and contents of the book.

2 The book jacket, if available, may describe the book.

3 Reading the table of contents and index of the book will give you important information about whether it will meet your information needs.

There are some guidelines that you can use to make a preliminary evaluation about the quality of a book.

1 What are the author's qualifications? Has the author published frequently on this topic?

2 If current information is important to you, has the book been published recently? Remember that there is a considerable length of time between a book's being written and its being available for sale.

3 Is this a second or later edition of the book? That a book has been revised, updated, and kept in print may be an indicator of its value.

4 Who published the book? The large publishing companies and university presses stake their reputations on the publication of quality books.

5 Does the book have up-to-date reference lists and bibliographies?

6 How have published book reviews evaluated the book?

7 In what country was the book published? If it was published in a country other than the United States, is its viewpoint relevant to the practice of nursing in the United States?

Publications by Professional Nursing Organizations

National nursing organizations are the source of many information resources of great importance to nursing. Many specialty nursing organizations, such as the Oncology Nurses Society, publish journals and other information resources. The American Nurses Association publishes books on nursing practice, education, and research; career issues; computers in nursing; quality improvement; nursing ethics; and other nursing topics. In collaboration with nursing specialty organizations, it publishes sets of professional nursing standards. It also publishes important policy statements and nursing white papers. A catalog of ANA information resources is available from American Nurses Publishing, 1-800-637-0323. Members of state nurses organizations receive a discounted price.

The National League for Nursing (NLN) is the other national organization publishing nursing resources. It publishes books on clinical topics, nursing history, nursing education, research and theory, and other areas of interest to nurses. A catalog can be obtained by calling 1-800-NOW-9NLN.

Government Documents

The U.S. Government is probably the largest publisher in the country. A wide variety of publications is available, ranging from statistical summaries to technical reports and popular consumer information. The Monthly Catalog of United States Government Publications, available in many libraries, indexes all of these publications by subject, author, and title. Many of these publications can be purchased. The U.S. Government Printing Office operates 24 bookstores around the country. You can also order the publications by writing to the U.S. Government Printing Office, Superintendent of Documents, Mail Stop: SSOP, Washington, DC 20402-9328, or by calling 1-202-783-3238. Your library may have some or all of the U.S. Government publications. Ask the librarian for assistance.

Journals

Probably the most up-to-date information is found in journals. A journal is published on a regular basis, such as monthly or quarterly, and contains articles related to a specific discipline or profession, such as nursing. Some nursing journals emphasize clinical practice, while others focus on nursing research, professional issues, or trends in the nursing profession.

Locating Journal Literature

Since it is too time consuming to check the tables of contents for all journal issues to find articles on a particular topic, periodical indexes list the articles by author, subject, or other category. These indexes are printed on a regular basis and/or are available for use on a computer. Computerized indexes are usually referred to as bibliographic databases. Print and computerized indexes will be described later in this guide.

Evaluating Journal Literature

As with books, a journal article may include information that is outdated, incorrect, or not relevant to your learning need. It is important to evaluate the information you read in any journal article. The questions you would ask yourself about a book, such as those listed above, are relevant to your evaluation of journal articles. Another guide to evaluating journal articles is discovering whether the article is published in a "peer reviewed" journal. Although the process varies among journals, peer review means that a manuscript submitted to a journal for publication is evaluated anonymously by one or more experts in the content area of the proposed article. The journal editor makes the decision to publish based on the judgments and recommendations of the reviewer(s). The journal masthead will indicate if the journal is peer reviewed.

LOCATING INFORMATION RESOURCES

Print Indexes

There are many print indexes to journal literature that nurses may use to find relevant articles. An index provides the basic elements of information that you need to locate an article. These

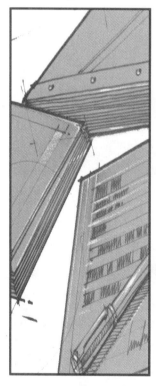

elements include the author and title of the article, the journal title, the volume and year, and the pages of the article. "Citation" or "bibliographic citation" are terms often used to describe this collection of elements. Those indexes which you may consult frequently are described below.

Cumulative Index to Nursing & Allied Health Literature® Print Index

This print index, published by Cinahl Information Systems, provides coverage of the literature in nursing and allied health. Virtually all English-language nursing journals are indexed along with publications from the American Nurses Association and the National League for Nursing. Foreign-language journals with English abstracts are also indexed. Primary journals in seventeen allied health disciplines are indexed, as well as selected journals in biomedicine and consumer health. In all, almost 1,100 serial publications are indexed. Cinahl also indexes selected healthcare books and book chapters, conference proceedings, nursing dissertations, and standards of professional practice. The print index is published as five bimonthly issues and an annual hardbound cumulation. Materials are indexed by author and subject.

International Nursing Index (INI)

The International Nursing Index is published quarterly by Lippincott-Raven Publishers in cooperation with the National Library of Medicine. It indexes almost 300 U.S. and international nursing journals and includes articles in English and foreign languages. In addition, it indexes nursing articles published in the biomedical and allied health journals indexed in Index Medicus and the HealthStar database. Articles are indexed by author and subject. There are also sections listing all new publications of the American Nurses' Association and the National League for Nursing, and new books received by Lippincott-Raven Publishers.

Index Medicus

Index Medicus is published by the National Library of Medicine and indexes English- and foreign-language journals in the biomedical sciences. It indexes journal articles by first author and three to five subject headings. It also indexes medical reviews which summarize the research of a particular subject area and provide extensive bibliographies. Index Medicus is published monthly, with annual cumulations. Abridged Index Medicus indexes the core English-language clinical journals most likely to be used by the medical practitioner.

Computerized Bibliographic Databases

While the print index provides only one information access point at a time, an electronic database allows you to search multiple data points simultaneously. The information available in the electronic format is more current because there is no printing and processing lag time. Many electronic databases have features that cannot be accessed in their print formats. However, some searches of a general nature may be more easily accomplished in the print format. Also, the print index is typically less costly for your library or health care agency than its electronic counterpart. However, as the information explosion continues into the 21st century and nurses become increasingly computer literate, computerized searching will provide a speedy, convenient, and focused approach to finding answers to nursing and health care questions.

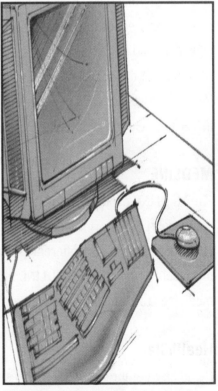

Computerized databases are produced in two formats. An online database is accessed by your computer via a modem. You can access the database directly, or through a contract or subscription with an online vendor. Your library may have such a subscription to one or more online databases. It is also possible to subscribe to online databases as an individual. The other format for computerized databases is CD-ROM. A CD-ROM (which stands for compact disc, read-only memory) is capable of storing vast amounts of information. If your library subscribes to the database in CD-ROM format, it will receive a new disc on a regular basis, often monthly, that will contain the updated database. Many databases are produced in both online and CD-ROM versions. The title of the database may vary depending on the version.

The computerized databases that you are most likely to use are described below. If you are doing a comprehensive or multidisciplinary literature search, it is important to use more than one database as each one has its own approach to indexing, even with the same article.

The CINAHL® Database

The computer version of the CUMULATIVE INDEX TO NURSING & ALLIED HEALTH LITERATURE® print index provides coverage from 1982 to the present. In addition to indexing the materials described above for the print index, the computerized version indexes educational software and audiovisual materials. In addition, abstracts are available for more than 700 journal titles, dissertations, educational software, and audiovisuals. Other features include indication of author affiliations and any research instruments used. The number of references in an article's bibliography is noted and the actual cited references are provided for articles from many journals. Seventeen journal subsets can help to narrow and refine the number of citations found. More information on the various features of the CINAHL database can be found later in this manual.

MEDLINE

The MEDLINE database is produced by the National Library of Medicine and is the computerized counterpart of the print indexes Index Medicus, International Nursing Index, and Index to Dental Literature. One major difference from the print version is that articles are indexed with many more subject headings. MEDLINE indexes English-and foreign-language journals in the areas of medicine, allied health, and the basic life sciences.

HealthStar

HealthStar comprehensively indexes materials in the nonclinical aspects of health care delivery.

Subject coverage includes health policy, health care, planning and administration, economics, health services research, and health care technology assessment. Materials indexed include journals, books, conference papers, and technical reports.

Educational Resources Information Center (ERIC)

The ERIC database, produced by the U.S. Office of Education, indexes literature in education and education-related areas. It indexes both published journals and unpublished reports. The unpublished reports are designated as "ERIC Documents" and are available from the ERIC Document Reproduction Service in print or microfiche formats (1-800-443-3742, 7420 Fullerton Rd., Suite 110, Springfield, VA 22153) or in large libraries in the microfiche format. ERIC is unique in the large amount of unpublished literature that it indexes; many of these documents contain valuable information. Areas of interest to nurses covered by ERIC include education of the handicapped and disadvantaged, early childhood education, and nursing education.

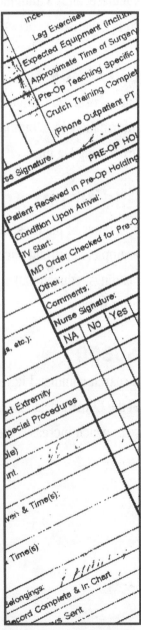

PsycINFO®

Produced by the American Psychological Association, PsycINFO is a computerized database that indexes journals, technical reports, dissertations, and other materials in all areas of psychology and the behavioral sciences. PsycINFO is the computerized version of the print index Psychological Abstracts, but the PsycINFO database indexes more materials than its print counterpart. PsycLIT® is a CD-ROM database that is a subset of PsycINFO. Another subset database is ClinPSYC®, intended to meet the needs of practicing clinicians in mental health settings.

Sociological Abstracts

Sociological Abstracts indexes the literature of sociology and related areas in the social, behavioral, and health sciences. Its coverage includes journals, dissertations, book abstracts and reviews, and conference proceedings abstracts. You will want to consult Sociological Abstracts if you are looking for information on the sociocultural aspects of illness and health.

PRINT INDEX vs. DATABASE: THE ELECTRONIC ADVANTAGE

An electronic database offers you flexibility, currency, additional access, speed, and convenience when searching for a topic.

Flexibility

A print index provides only one information access point at a time, whereas an electronic database allows multifaceted searching. The retrieval of citations becomes an efficient and comprehensive process.

Currency

The information available in an electronic format is more current due to monthly updates. Information in a bimonthly or quarterly print index is not as timely due to the printing and processing lag time.

Additional Access

A number of features can be accessed in a bibliographic database but not in a print index. For example, important parts of the CINAHL® database, such as abstracts, full text, minor (non-print) headings, educational software, cited references, and grant information, are not included in the print version.

Speed

A search command keyed in will retrieve material for a number of years – seventeen in the case of the CINAHL database. In the print index the searcher has to conduct separate searches for each year, which increases the time it takes to conduct the search.

ETHICAL ISSUES IN THE USE OF INFORMATION

Once you have located information, it is important to keep certain ethical considerations in mind in the use of that information. Other than the information contained in U.S. Government publications, which is in the public domain, most information found in the resources described in this guide is protected by copyright laws.

Another important ethical consideration in the use of information is the concept of plagiarism, the act of presenting someone else's work as your own. If you quote directly from an information source, quotation marks must be used and the source of the quotation documented. If you are paraphrasing the information that you have located, you must give credit to the original author or source.

References

1. Gee, E.G., Breivik, P.S. Libraries and learning. ERIC Document ED284593, 1987.

2. Fingerhut, E.R. A probe of library references, 2d rev. ed. Claremont, CA: The Paige Press, 1992.

Searching the Literature for Information

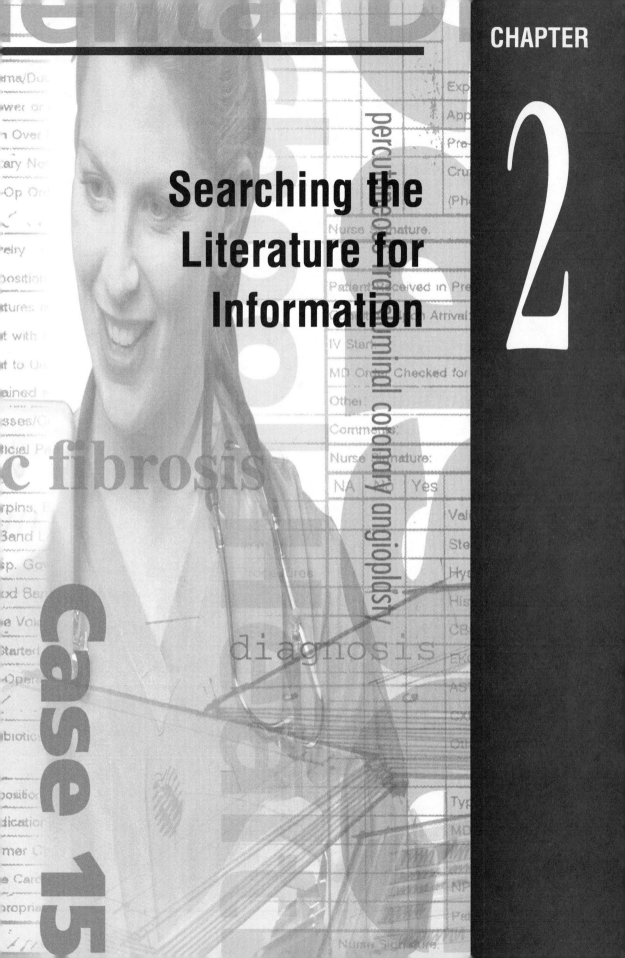

he concept of an index is one with which we are all familiar. Indexes classify and categorize a certain body of information and allow us to find that information most pertinent to our specific learning need. Let's use a clinical example to think about a familiar index – the index to a book. Imagine that you are the leader of a support group for nurses who work with terminally ill children. Recently, the group sessions have been characterized by many periods of silence. To enhance your skills as a group leader you want to learn more about silence in groups and how to respond to it. Your supervisor has told you about a book for nurses on leading groups, and by using the book catalog, you locate the book, The Nurse as Group Leader, 3rd. ed., by Carolyn Chambers Clark.

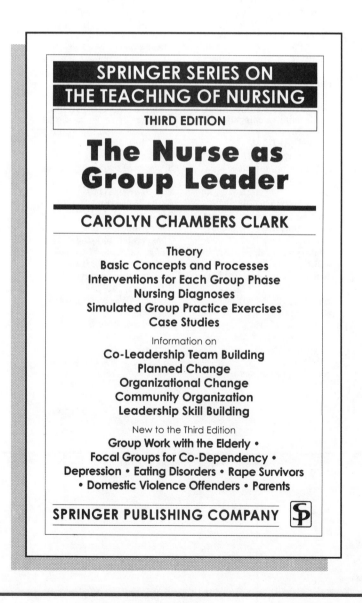

SPRINGER SERIES ON THE TEACHING OF NURSING

THIRD EDITION

The Nurse as Group Leader

CAROLYN CHAMBERS CLARK

Theory
Basic Concepts and Processes
Interventions for Each Group Phase
Nursing Diagnoses
Simulated Group Practice Exercises
Case Studies

Information on
Co-Leadership Team Building
Planned Change
Organizational Change
Community Organization
Leadership Skill Building

New to the Third Edition
Group Work with the Elderly •
Focal Groups for Co-Dependency •
Depression • Eating Disorders • Rape Survivors
• Domestic Violence Offenders • Parents

SPRINGER PUBLISHING COMPANY SP

Subject Searching

You turn to the back of the book to consult the index and find a listing for silence.

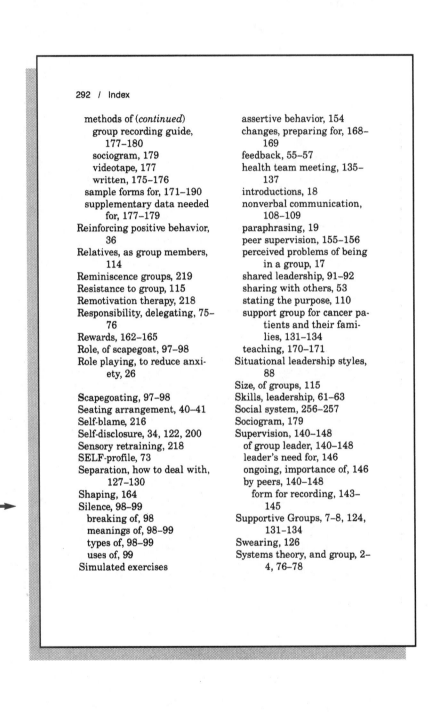

You go to that section of the book, read the information on silence, and decide to talk to a fellow group leader about implementing some of the suggested approaches.

98 / The Nurse as Group Leader

is it possible you have some critical feelings toward me, too?"

To deal effectively with scapegoating, the leader must be willing to accept anger. The leader needs to be able to accept verbal anger, resentment, or disappointment without trying to change the subject, to comply with unrealistic group demands, or to retaliate in subtle ways. By accepting group anger appropriately, the leader can help the group to learn that authority figures are human and should not be expected to meet everyone's needs, but that this does not necessarily mean that they are punitive or nonaccepting of others' feelings.

SILENCE

The ability to use silence effectively is a learned skill. Some silences are useful to group movement, others are not. Silence can be a group or an individual phenomenon. In either case, silence can have a number of meanings. Individual silence may mean that the person is holding back information or self in order to punish the group or the leader, may fear displeasing others, is in agreement, or is trying to escape talking because he is anxious.

When silence pervades the group early, it is often used to conceal that group members are anxious and unsure of what to do. Those who are least comfortable with silence will usually speak first. Often those who break silences do so because they think they are responsible for keeping the group moving. *Sad silences* may follow discussion of separation, death, or ending of the group. *Angry silences* follow angry interchanges and may be clues to hidden hostility or resentment that can decrease group movement. *Thoughtful silences* can occur after an especially relevant interchange.

In many groups there is a tendency to assume that the leader should break silences, and this may be most comfortable for an inexperienced leader. In general, it is best for the leader not to break silences unless they appear to be

Reprinted with permission

Bibliographic Databases

Just as a book uses an index to help you find specific information within the book, indexing is used by bibliographic databases to help you locate journal articles and other resources.

Most bibliographic databases have developed a list of subject headings that is used as a predetermined index to all of the journal articles and other materials covered by that database. This list of subject headings is also referred to as a thesaurus or a controlled vocabulary.

Subject heading lists aid in the selection of useful search terms because they provide leads from one subject heading to a more preferred subject heading, and also indicate relationships between terms. The following section describes the techniques of subject searching for one specific database: the CINAHL® database.

CINAHL Subject Searching

The CINAHL Subject Headings List (or "yellow pages") is the key to effective searching of the CINAHL database. It includes all nursing and allied health subject headings and cross-references arranged in three formats: Alphabetic, Tree Structure, and Permuted Structure.

Think about your search topic and make sure you have broken it down into its most basic components. For a more detailed explanation of the Thesaurus, consult the *"SEE THE CITES WITH CINAHL®"* instructional CD-ROM (directions on page 246) accompanying this guide, or contact Cinahl Information Systems at 1-800-959-7167 for the VHS tape.

Alphabetic Section

Start with the Alphabetic List of the "yellow pages." Look up your topic to see if it is a valid heading. (Valid headings will appear in all capitals.) If it is not, a "see" reference may lead you to the appropriate heading for your topic. For example, when you look up *Cancer Nursing*, the cross-reference "see Oncologic Nursing" tells you that articles on this topic appear under the heading *Oncologic Nursing* and not under *Cancer Nursing*.

Scope notes and indexing notes clarify the usage of many subject headings that might be useful. When you look up *Oncologic Nursing*, you will find an indexing note indicating the precoordinated heading *Pediatric Oncology Nursing*.

The following sample entries from the Alphabetic List show you the information that is included about subject headings. The notes that follow the two examples explain the various features.

Sample Entries from the Alphabetic List

Sample 1

A plus(+) sign indicates narrower terms are available

Valid Subject Heading —— **FETAL MONITORING**

$E1.249.259.400+   E1.621.390+

Year: 1983 ———— *Date*

Dollar ($) sign indicates different position in the MeSH Tree Structures

Physiologic or biochemical monitoring of the fetus. Usually done during labor and may be in conjunction with monitoring of uterine activity. May also be prenatal as when the mother is undergoing surgery. FETAL MONITORING, ELECTRONIC is also available. —— *Scope Note*

see also FETAL MONITORING (IOWA NIC) • FETAL MOVEMENT • HEART RATE, FETAL —— *"See also" Reference*

"x" symbol —— x   Fetal Scalp Sampling • Monitoring, Fetal
"XX" symbol —— XX   LABOR • SIGNAL PROCESSING, COMPUTER ASSISTED

FETAL MONITORING, ELECTRONIC

$E1.249.259.400.395+ $E1.621.390.395+
Year: 1990

Before 1990 see under FETAL MONITORING.

x   Electronic Fetal Monitoring

Fetal Monitoring, Home see HOME FETAL MONITORING —— *"See" Reference*

Sample 2

BLOOD LOSS, SURGICAL

C23.542.100   C23.612.100
Year: 1991

Loss of blood during surgery. For blood loss following surgery, related or unrelated to the surgical wound, see HEMORRHAGE, POSTOPERATIVE. For /therapy or /prevention and control, use HEMOSTASIS, SURGICAL. —— *Scope Note may explain use of subheadings*

Before 1991 see under HEMORRHAGE; POSTOPERATIVE COMPLICATIONS. —— *History Note*

see also HEMOSTASIS, SURGICAL

x   Surgical Blood Loss

Notes on Samples

Subject Headings

Valid CINAHL subject headings are printed in capital letters.

Cross-References

"See" references refer from terms not used to valid CINAHL subject headings:
Fetal Monitoring, Home see HOME FETAL MONITORING.

Tree Numbers

Each subject heading is followed by one or more alphanumeric codes (tree numbers) which direct you to the place in the Tree Structures where the subject heading is to be found (see below).

Date

The date identifies which year a term was added as a subject heading.

Scope Note

The scope note provides a brief definition of headings that may be unclear and/or explains the use of subheadings.

The History Note

The history note explains where to find information on that topic in previous years.

See Also References

"See also" references indicate related CINAHL headings that do not appear in the same tree.

x and XX Symbols

The x symbol listed under a valid heading indicates a reference from an expression not itself used as a heading. The XX symbol indicates a related or broader subject heading from which a see also reference is made.

Tree Structures and Permuted Section

The Tree Structures list all CINAHL headings in a subject hierarchy which shows the relationship between broader and narrower terms. Consult the Permuted List if you cannot locate an appropriate subject heading in the Alphabetic List. Every significant word appearing in a CINAHL heading or cross-reference is listed here alphabetically.

A further description of the Tree Structures and Permuted Section of the Subject Heading List is found in the Advance Concepts of Searching section in this book.

Subject Heading Lists for Other Databases

Most databases have a published list of subject headings that is used when indexing all literature.

MEDLINE

- *Medical Subject Headings (MeSH) - Annotated Alphabetical List*, 1998. National Library of Medicine. 1997.
- *Medical Subject Headings - Tree Structures*, 1998. National Library of Medicine. 1997.
- *Permuted Medical Subject Headings*, 1998. National Library of Medicine. 1997.

ERIC

Thesaurus of ERIC Descriptors, 13th edition. The Oryx Press. 1995.

PSYCINFO

Thesaurus of Psychological Index Terms, Eighth Edition. American Psychological Association. 1997.

SOCIOLOGICAL ABSTRACTS

Thesaurus of Sociological Indexing Terms, Fourth Edition. Sociological Abstracts, Inc. 1996.

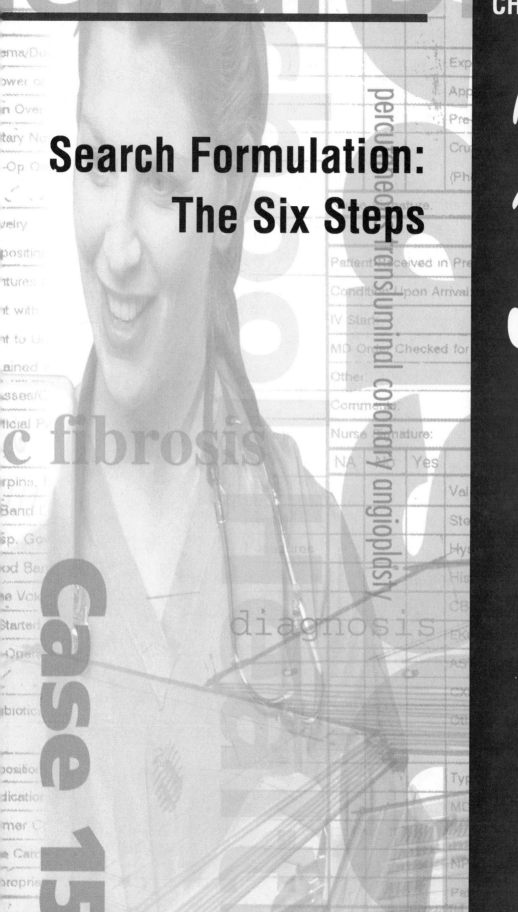

Search Formulation:
The Six Steps

ne of the most important aspects of searching the literature is formulating the exact strategy that you will use to obtain the information you want from the database. The following six steps will help you in your planning. These six steps will be used to guide you through the case studies later in this manual.

1 Plan your search strategy ahead of time

You will save time if you think through your topic and decide what focus you want your search to take.

2 Break down your search topic into components

Suppose you wish to find information on the nursing assessment of alcoholism. Remember to include synonyms or related terms. The components of your search would be alcoholism and nursing assessment.

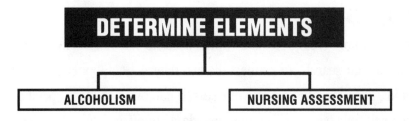

Sometimes the terms you have thought of for your search will be subject headings in the database's subject heading list (often called a thesaurus), and sometimes they won't.

3 Check for terms in a subject heading list

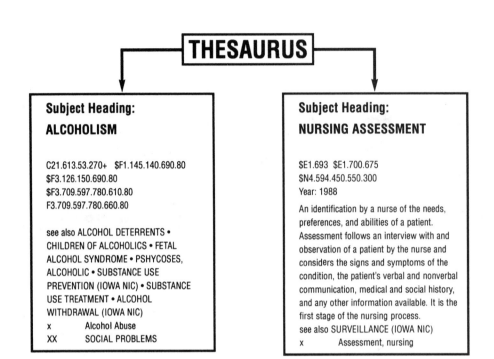

THESAURUS

Subject Heading:

ALCOHOLISM

C21.613.53.270+ $F1.145.140.690.80
$F3.126.150.690.80
$F3.709.597.780.610.80
F3.709.597.780.660.80

see also ALCOHOL DETERRENTS •
CHILDREN OF ALCOHOLICS • FETAL
ALCOHOL SYNDROME • PSHYCOSES,
ALCOHOLIC • SUBSTANCE USE
PREVENTION (IOWA NIC) • SUBSTANCE
USE TREATMENT • ALCOHOL
WITHDRAWAL (IOWA NIC)
x   Alcohol Abuse
XX   SOCIAL PROBLEMS

Subject Heading:

NURSING ASSESSMENT

$E1.693 $E1.700.675
$N4.594.450.550.300
Year: 1988

An identification by a nurse of the needs,
preferences, and abilities of a patient.
Assessment follows an interview with and
observation of a patient by the nurse and
considers the signs and symptoms of the
condition, the patient's verbal and nonverbal
communication, medical and social history,
and any other information available. It is the
first stage of the nursing process.
see also SURVEILLANCE (IOWA NIC)
x   Assessment, nursing

4 Select operators

The term "operator" refers to the word used to connect different or synonymous
components of your search. To connect the two different components of your search topic,
use the "and" operator. This makes your search narrower or more specific. The results of
your search will only have records that include *Alcoholism* "and" *Nursing Assessment* as
subject headings.

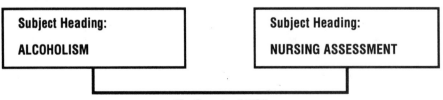

Subject Heading:

ALCOHOLISM

Subject Heading:

NURSING ASSESSMENT

Use Operator "AND"

The "or" operator can be used to connect synonymous or related terms. This broadens your search. In the example below "or" was used to connect synonymous textwords and broader headings to retrieve material before 1989.

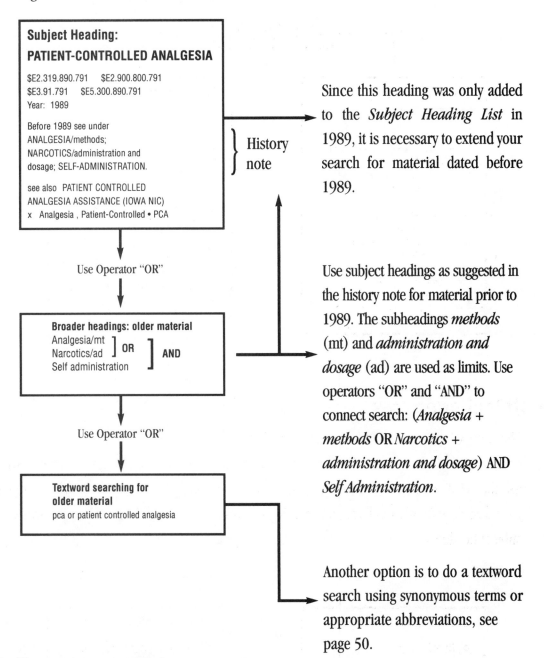

Since this heading was only added to the *Subject Heading List* in 1989, it is necessary to extend your search for material dated before 1989.

Use subject headings as suggested in the history note for material prior to 1989. The subheadings *methods* (mt) and *administration and dosage* (ad) are used as limits. Use operators "OR" and "AND" to connect search: (*Analgesia + methods* OR *Narcotics + administration and dosage*) AND *Self Administration*.

Another option is to do a textword search using synonymous terms or appropriate abbreviations, see page 50.

5 Run your search

6 View the results

Remember these six formulation steps as they will be used in the Case Studies Section in this manual.

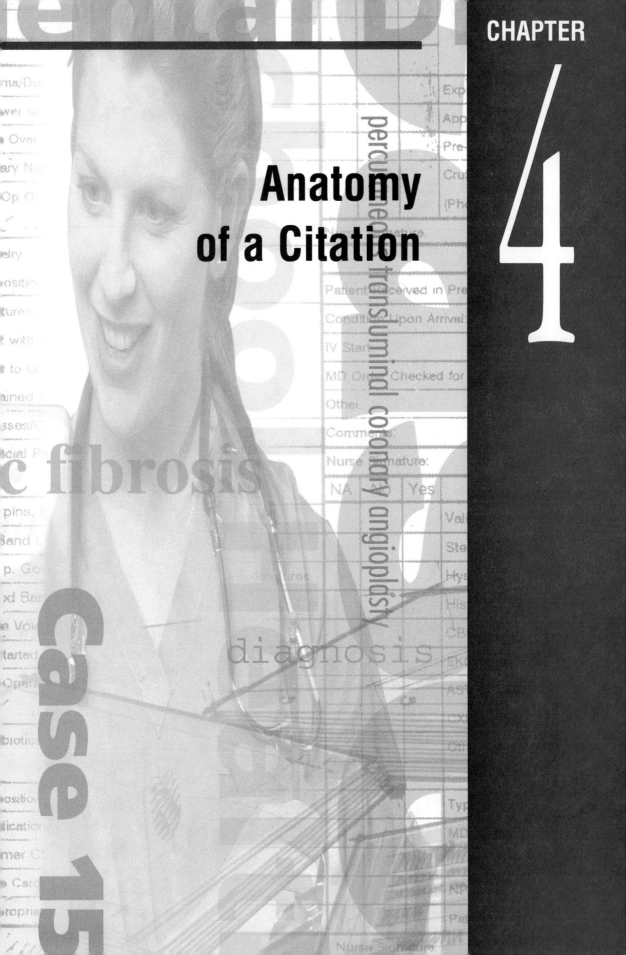

CHAPTER

4

Anatomy of a Citation

*W*hat follows are examples of records that you may find in your search for information on a topic. The information in each record is broken up into "fields." Each field is named and contains information pertinent to the named field. For example, you will find the author(s) listed in the author field, English listed in the language field. All fields are searchable. The record as a whole enables you to decide whether you need the journal article, book, etc., to meet your learning needs. You are given sufficient information to help you locate the item in a library. The notes that follow the examples explain the various fields.

Journal Record

Accession No.:	1996019336
Author:	Birenbaum LK. Stewart BJ. Phillips DS.
Author Affil:	Walter Cancer Institute and Indiana University School of Nursing, Indianapolis, IN
Title:	Health status of bereaved parents
Publication Yr:	1996
Source:	NURS RES 1996 Mar-Apr; 45(2): 105-9 (27 ref)
Full Jrnl Name:	Nursing Research
Journal Title:	NURS RES
Language:	English (EN)
Journal Subset:	Core-Nursing (CN). Nursing (NU). Peer-Reviewed (PR). USA (US).
ISSN:	0029-6562
Medline Number:	96186015
Instrumentation:	Duke-UNC Health Profile (Duke-UNC)
Serial ID:	N35180000
Pub Type:	Journal-Article (JNL). Research (RES). Tables-Charts (TCS).
Major Heading:	Health-Status. Parents. Bereavement. Death -- In-Infancy-and-Childhood (IIC). Childhood-Neoplasms – Psychosocial-Factors (PF).
Minor Heading:	Funding-Source. Prospective-Studies. Coefficient-Alpha. Questionnaires. Confidence-Intervals. Convenience-Sample. Repeated-Measures. Analysis-of-Variance. Interviews...
Abstract:	Forty-seven mothers and 33 fathers, representing 48 families, participated in a prospective longitudinal study of the effects on family members of a child's...
References:	Ahmed PI, Coelho GV. Toward a new definition of health: psychosocial dimensions. New York: Plenum; 1979. Baumer JH, Wadsworth J, Taylor B. Family recovery after death of a child. Archives of Disease in Childhood 1988; 63: 942-947...
Grant Info:	Department of Health and Human Services, Division of Nursing and National Center for Nursing Research Grants #RO1 NU00912 and #RO1 NU00912 02S1
Updatd Code:	9606

Book Record

Accession No.: 1994198336
Author: Bullough B. Bullough VL.
Author Affil: SUNY Coll, Buffalo NY.
Title: Nursing issues for the nineties and beyond
Publication Yr: 1994
Source: Springer Publ (New York, NY) **1994 (240 p) (54 ref)
Language: English
ISBN: 0-8261-8050-7
Pub Type: Book (BKS)
Major Heading: Nursing-Practice--United States
Nursing-as-a-Profession--United States
Minor Heading: United States
Nursing-as-a-Profession/Trends (TD)
Publisher: Springer Publishing Co.
Update Code: 9411

Book Chapter Record

Accession No.: 1994198349
Author: Bullough B. Bullough VL.
Author Affil: SUNY Coll, Buffalo NY
Title: Opportunities for specialty nursing practice IN:
Nursing issues for the nineties and beyond (Bullough B et al)
Publication Yr: 1994
Source: Springer Publ (New York, NY) ** 1994 (pp 9-21) (31 ref)
Language: English (EN)
ISBN: 0-8261-8050-7
Pub Type: Book-Chapter (BKC)
Major Heading: Specialties, Nursing
Minor Heading: Nursing-Organizations.
Nursing-as-a-Profession--United States.
United-States.
Advanced-Practice-Nurses.
Publisher: Springer Publishing Co.
Update Code: 9411

Research Instrument Record

Accession No.: 1996020627

Author: Robinson BC.

Title: Caregiver Strain Index (CSI)

Source: Department of Family & Community Medicine,
University of California, San Francisco,
500 Parnassus Avenue, MU-3 East, Box 0900,
San Francisco, CA 94143 (1 p) (2 ref)

Language: English (EN)

Pub Type: Research-Instrument (RIN). Questionnaire (QUE).

Major Heading: Caregiver-Burden--Evaluation (EV).
Psychosocial-Aspects-of-Illness -- Evaluation (EV).
Caregivers--Psychosocial-Factors (PF).

Minor Heading: Coefficient-Alpha. Construct-Validity. Interviews.

Abstract: The CSI is an interviewer-administered 13-item instrument designed as a screening procedure to detect strain in individuals acting in caregiving...

Description: YEAR DEVELOPED: 1979-1983
PURPOSE: A screening procedure to detect strain...
VARIABLES OF INTEREST: Responses to thirteen...
ORIGINAL POPULATION: A sample of 85 spouses,...
QUESTION FORMAT: The interview schedule is...
ADMINISTRATION: Interviewer-administered in 10...
SCORING: Affirmative answers are totaled; the...
PSYCHOMETRICS: A reliability coefficient of .86...
HOW TO OBTAIN: Questions regarding ...
COPYRIGHT OWNER: The Gerontological Society...
MODIFICATIONS: None
Description Copyright (c) 1996, Cinahl Information Systems

Full Text: CAREGIVER STRAIN INDEX
I am going to read a list of things which other people...

References: Robinson BC. Validation of a Caregiver Strain Index.
Journal of Gerontology 1983; 38(3): 344-8.
Robinson BC, Thurner M. Taking care of aged parents:
a family cycle transition. The Gerontologist 1979;...

Update Code: 9606

Notes on Records

Remember that all fields are searchable.

Accession Number

Cinahl assigns a unique ten-digit number to each record in the database. These numbers will help you locate specific citations.

Author

Don't forget this field for those times you want to find material by specific authors – perhaps a journal article by a colleague, instructor, nurse theorist, etc. The personal author's last name is followed by one or more initials, up to three (e.g., Saba VK).

Corporate Author

Corporate author names are listed as they appear in the document: US Public Health Services. Agency for Health Care Policy and Research. Try to find out what publications your school has authored.

Author Affiliation

The business/institutional address for the first author is listed. If you need to determine which organization is involved in certain research do a textword search in this field. For example, in the sample journal record on page 33, the Walter Cancer Institute was associated with research on the health status of bereaved parents.

Title

Need to find a specific article, book, pamphlet, dissertation, or audiovisual? Look in the title field!

Series Title

Series titles for books, pamphlets, and journals are included in this field.

Publication Year

Your assignment is to find material for the last five years – the publication year will help you determine the currency of the material you retrieve in your search.

Source

The source field for journal records includes the abbreviation of the journal title, publication date, volume and issue number, pagination, and number of references. In book, audiovisual, and software records the publishers, producers, or distributors are identified. This information is essential to locating the item in a library.

Full Journal Name

The full journal title is listed in this field.

Language

The language of each document is indicated. If you want only English documents remember to limit your search to English.

Review

The review field will indicate where you can find a review of the journal article, book, audiovisual, or pamphlet you retrieved in your search.

ISBN

International Standard Book Numbers are included in the database to help you identify a title universally.

ISSN

Most journal titles in the database are assigned International Standard Serial Numbers to help you identify a title universally.

Serial ID

National Library of Medicine's nine-digit serial identifier numbers will help your librarian identify journal titles when ordering articles for you from another library.

Journal Subsets

Journal subsets are listed in this field to identify subject category, country in which the journal is published, and/or whether it is peer reviewed.

Publication Type

You are asked to find five research articles published in peer reviewed nursing journals: you need to limit (detailed on pages 42-43) using subsets (nursing, peer reviewed) and publication type (research). Check this field to see if you retrieved what you searched for!

Research Instruments

Research instruments, clinical assessment tools, and psychological tests used in the research study you retrieved are listed in this field.

Grant Information

When a study or document has been funded the information pertaining to the grant or partial grant will be included in this field.

Major Heading

Major headings indicate the focus of the document indexed.

Minor Heading

Minor headings indicate that only a small part of the document covers the topic you searched.

Terms in Process

This field includes subject headings that are being considered for inclusion in next year's CINAHL Subject Heading List. Remember that the Subject Heading List is updated annually.

Abstract

Author and CINAHL abstracts are usually available to help you decide whether a document is appropriate for your assignment.

References

References cited at the end of journal articles in selected nursing and allied health journals are available. This reference list may be a useful additional bibliography on your topic.

Medline Number

The National Library of Medicine's unique identifier number has been added to the CINAHL®

database. These numbers will assist your librarian in ordering journal articles from another library if they are not in your library's journal collection.

Entry Month

A four-digit code is assigned to each record indicating the year and month the record was added to the index (e.g., 9701 for January of 1997).

Table of Contents

This field lists the title, author (if available), and page numbers of items that are part of a whole document, such as "blurbs" in a regular column in a journal, book chapters in a book, abstracts/articles in proceedings, etc. The table of contents gives you a better idea of the format of the document you are trying to locate.

Description

Cinahl provides its own descriptions of research instruments and websites.

Full Text

Forty-one state nursing journals and selected government publications (practice guidelines, patient education material, etc.), nurse practice acts, standards of nursing practice, and research instruments are available in full text. Cinahl provides its own clinical innovations, accreditation records, legal cases, and drug records.

Image

Critical paths and research instruments are available as images. The PDF file number is provided to help you locate the image.

Search Strategy: Broad vs. Narrow

To decide if your search should be broad or narrow, you need to address the following questions:

1 What is the purpose of the search and how do you plan to use the results of the search – is it to answer a specific clinical question or is it for a research paper where a comprehensive search of the topic is necessary?

2 How many articles do you need to retrieve – do you need an extensive bibliography or only a few references?

3 Do you wish to include only those articles with a major focus on your topic or do you want related material as well?

Explosions

The Explode command can be used with CINAHL or MeSH (MEDLINE) headings to retrieve the heading and all the specific terms under it, i.e., to explode a subject heading is to retrieve any specific aspects of the more general topic. You explode a topic if all aspects of the topic are wanted. If you only want the specific topic do not explode.

Subject Heading	Documents	
Critical Care Nursing	6711	
Burn Nursing	267	Exploding Critical Care Nursing will retrieve all documents shown here
Coronary Care Nursing	814	
Pediatric Critical Care Nursing	758	
Neonatal Intensive Care Nursing	505	

In a broad search, the number of search formulations or concepts is reduced and the number of articles retrieved increased. Restrictions or limitations such as language, publication year, or document type are kept to a minimum.

In a narrow search, the search formulations or concepts are more complex. Fewer articles will be retrieved and the number of articles can be further limited by restricting the descriptors to major headings; by adding topical, geographic, or age subheadings; or by limiting to specific document types.

Selecting the Appropriate Database

Once you have formulated your search strategy, you need to select the database(s) with the most comprehensive coverage for your search. For a comprehensive literature search you should search all appropriate databases using all the search options available in each. Only in this way can you retrieve from one database the relevant references that others may have missed.

The points you will want to consider when selecting a bibliographic database are:

What subjects are covered in the search and which bibliographic database focuses on those subject areas specifically?

What type of resource (journal, book, audiovisual, computer software, etc.) contains material on the subject and what database covers the format required?

Does the database cover the years required? What is the size of the database? How often is the database updated? Are journals included on a cover-to-cover basis or are only selected references added to the database?

How heavily may a searcher rely on the subject heading list (controlled vocabulary a.k.a. thesaurus) of a database?

What kind of indexing is provided by the database? Is it specific and in-depth, or is broader coverage provided?

Which database allows you to find answers to specific questions? *A database with good access points (fields with author or journal names, or information indicating where a book has been reviewed or when a research instrument has been used in a research article, etc.) allows you to find these answers.*

Does the database allow you to narrow the search strategy?

Answers to these questions about the CINAHL® database will be found in Appendix 1.

Modifying Search Strategy

Once you have selected your database and conducted your search you may need to modify your search strategy if it produces too many citations (often referred to as "hits"). The following section lists seven strategies for modifying a search topic using the CINAHL® database. Many databases have similar options that you can use.

Major Subject Headings

The most popular way of modifying a search strategy is by limiting to major terms. If you select a major subject heading on the topic you have chosen you will get articles specifically on your topic (also referred to as "restrict to focus").

Subheadings

There are 67 subheadings (see Appendix 2 for complete list) that can be linked to CINAHL main headings. CINAHL main headings can be modified by the addition of subheadings to provide more specific access. For example, if you are seeking information on the psychosocial aspects of AIDS, you would use the subject heading *Acquired Immunodeficiency Syndrome* and the subheading *psychosocial factors*. Not all subheadings can be used with all main headings: for example, the subheading *prevention and control* is meaningless linked to the main heading *Nursing Protocols*.

Tertiary Subheadings

Two other groups of headings are available – population groups and geographics (see Appendix 3 for list of population groups). Like topical subheadings, tertiary headings can be used to limit your subject even further: *Substance Abuse – in adolescence – United States*

Document (Publication) Types

Document types are assigned for every CINAHL citation (see Appendix 4 for complete list). There are three reasons for assigning a document type:

1 To represent the type of publication being indexed, e.g., journal, book, book chapter, audiovisual, pamphlet, pamphlet chapter, software, dissertation, critical path, or research instrument: Typical question: **Find a *book* on Alzheimer's Disease**.

2 To describe the format of the individual article being indexed, e.g., editorial, research, review, overall, etc.:
Typical question: **Find a *research* article on breast feeding**.

3 To indicate the presence of some special data, e.g., exam questions, care plan, questionnaire, tracings, diagnostic images, algorithm, cartoon, tables/charts, forms, etc.: Typical question: **Find a *critical path* on ventilation**.

Journal Subsets

Seventeen journal subsets have been created to help refine your search strategy.

1 Africa

2 Allied Health

3 Alternative/Complementary Therapies

4 Asia

5 Australia & New Zealand

6 Biomedical

7 Canada

8 Consumer Health

9 Core Nursing - assigned to all articles from nursing journals recommended in the "Brandon-Hill List," i.e., the premier journals in the field. All journals in this subset are included in the nursing subset. This subset is particularly valuable for quality filtering.

10 Europe

11 Health Services Administration

12 Information Science

13 Mexico & Central/South America

14 Nursing

15 Peer Reviewed - assigned to all articles from peer reviewed journals. Individual articles retrieved may NOT have been peer reviewed although the journals they appear in require it of MOST items published. This subset is particularly valuable for quality filtering.

16 UK & Ireland is assigned to all articles from journals published in England, Scotland, Wales, Northern Ireland, and the Republic of Ireland (Eire).

17 USA

Publication Year

If you are interested in only the most current information on a topic, you may want to limit your search to the last year or two.

Language

Non-English publications are included in the database. The search can be restricted to a specific language.

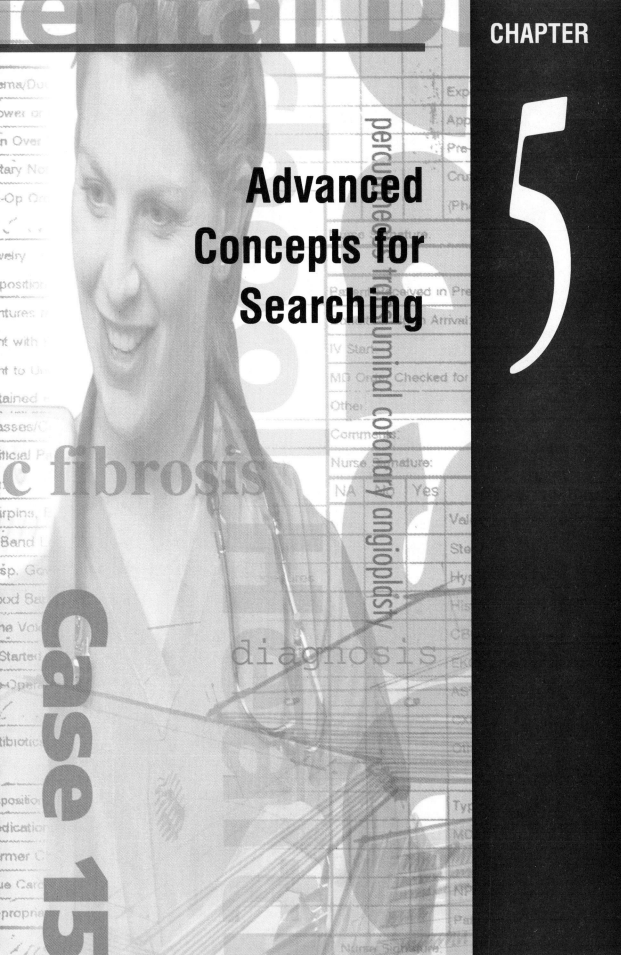

Advanced Concepts for Searching

*t*his section presents some advanced concepts for searching the literature using the CINAHL®
database. It includes a description of the Tree Structure and Permuted List sections of the *Subject
Heading List* and descriptions of additional access points.

Tree Structures

The second section of the CINAHL Subject Heading List is the Tree Structures. The Tree Structures
list all CINAHL headings in a subject hierarchy which shows the relationship between broader and
narrower terms. Alphanumeric codes ("tree numbers") from the Alphabetic List guide you to the
appropriate trees (G2 & N2 for *Oncologic Nursing*). Careful use of the Tree Structures can also
help you to select the most appropriate heading(s).

Consult the Tree Structures to select the most appropriate and specific heading(s) related to your
topic. This is important since indexers always assign the most specific subject headings available.
Refer to the sample entry from the Tree Structures below. If you are looking for articles on
Pediatric Oncology Nursing, you must search under that heading; articles specific to pediatrics
will not also appear under the more general term *Oncologic Nursing*.

ONCOLOGIC NURSING	N2.421.533.520.805+	G2.478.675
PEDIATRIC ONCOLOGY NURSING	N2.421.533.520.805.745	G2.478.675

Tree Categories

The trees are composed of 16 broad categories:

- A   Anatomy
- B   Organisms
- C   Diseases
- D   Chemicals and Drugs
- E   Analytical, Diagnostic, and Therapeutic Techniques and Equipment
- F   Psychiatry and Psychology
- G   Biological Sciences

H   Physical Sciences

I   Anthropology, Education, Sociology and Social Phenomena

J   Technology, Industry, Agriculture, Food

K   Liberal Arts

L   Information Science and Communication

M   Named Groups

N   Health Care

P   Classification Systems

Z   Geographic Names

Most of the trees are further divided into subcategories, e.g., A7=Anatomy – Cardiovascular System. CINAHL subject headings in each sub-category are in a subject hierarchy showing the relationship between broader and narrower terms. The following sample entry from the Tree Structures further illustrates the hierarchical relations among subject headings.

Sample Entry from the Tree Structures

	Tree Number	Cross-Reference Tree Numbers indicate other tree locations		
ADVANCED PRACTICE NURSES	$N2.350.645.630.200.108+	M1.526.485		
CLINICAL NURSE SPECIALISTS	$N2.350.645.630.200.108.205	M1.526.485		
NURSE ANESTHETISTS	$N2.350.645.630.200.108.600	M1.526.485	N2.350.645	N2.350.675
NURSE MIDWIVES	$N2.350.645.630.200.108.620	M1.526.485	M1.526.485	N2.350.645
NURSE PRACTITIONERS	$N2.350.645.630.200.108.640+	M1.526.485		
ACUTE NURSE PRACTITIONERS	$N2.350.645.630.200.108.640.105	M1.526.485		
ADULT NURSE PRACTITIONERS	$N2.350.645.630.200.108.640.115	M1.526.485		
FAMILY NURSE PRACTITIONERS	$N2.350.645.630.200.108.640.305	M1.526.485		
GERONTOLOGIC NURSE PRACTITIONERS	$N2.350.645.630.200.108.640.415	M1.526.485	M1.526.485	N2.350.645
OB-GYN NURSE PRACTITIONERS	$N2.350.645.630.200.108.640.590	M1.526.485		
PEDIATRIC NURSE PRACTITIONERS	$N2.350.645.630.200.108.640.630+	M1.526.485	M1.526.485	N2.350.645
NEONATAL NURSE PRACTITIONERS	$N2.350.645.630.200.108.640.630.590	M1.526.485	M1.526.485	N2.350.645
NURSE PSYCHOTHERAPISTS	$N2.350.645.630.200.108.650	M1.526.485	M1.526.485	M1.526.485
CASE MANAGERS	$N2.350.645.630.200.180	M1.526.180	M1.526.485	M1.526.485
FACULTY, NURSING	$N2.350.645.630.200.325	I2.463.473	M1.526.339	1.526.485

Notes on Sample

Tree Numbers: In the Tree Structures each subject heading is followed by a tree number that indicates its position in the hierarchy. The subject heading may also be followed by one or more additional numbers in smaller type that indicate other tree locations for the same heading. A plus (+) sign at the end of the number indicates that a more specific subject heading is available.

Permuted

The third section of the CINAHL Subject Heading List is the Permuted List. Consult the Permuted List if you cannot locate an appropriate subject heading in the Alphabetic List. Every significant word appearing within a CINAHL heading or cross-reference is listed here alphabetically. It can be a very powerful tool when only one word of a heading is known. Once a term is located, refer to the Alphabetic Section to check how it is used.

The Permuted List also provides a link between headings and cross-references which might be related but which do not necessarily appear together in either the Alphabetic List or the Tree Structures.

Sample Entry from the Permuted List

EDUCATION, POST-RN	Subject Heading
EDUCATION, PREMEDICAL	Cross-Reference
Alphabetic Listing — **Education,** Problem-Based *see* PROBLEM-BASED LEARNING	
Education, Professional, Retraining *see* REFRESHER COURSES	
Education Providers, Continuing *see* CONTINUING EDUCATION PROVIDERS	
EDUCATION, RADIOLOGICAL TECHNOLOGY	
EDUCATION, RESEARCH	
EDUCATION, RESPIRATORY THERAPY	
EDUCATION, SOCIAL WORK	
EDUCATION, SPECIAL	
EDUCATION, SPEECH-LANGUAGE PATHOLOGY	
Education Studies *see* EDUCATION RESEARCH	
EDUCATION, SURGICAL TECHNOLOGY	
EDUCATION, THEORY BASED	
Education, Vocational see VOCATIONAL EDUCATION	
Emergency Medical Services **Education** *see* EDUCATION, EMERGENCY MEDICAL SERVICES	

Notes on Sample

Every significant word appearing in a CINAHL heading or cross-reference is listed alphabetically in the Permuted List.

Each entry includes the word in bold print in uppercase if it is a subject heading or in uppercase and lowercase if it is a cross-reference.

Once a term is located, refer to the Alphabetic List to check how it is used.

OTHER ACCESS POINTS

If subject headings do not answer your information needs, consider using the specific information in other fields (other access points). There are three categories of access points available in the CINAHL® database: subject focused, bibliographic, and value added.

1 The subject focus fields which can be used as access points are title, series title, abstract, full text, and terms in process.

2 The bibliographic fields which can be used as access points are author, corporate author, cited references, accession numbers, table of contents, and source information.

3 The value-added fields (fields which add more information to the basic bibliographic record) are those providing information on instrumentation; author affiliations; ISBN, ISSN, and UMI, numbers; pamphlet numbers; serial identifier numbers; grant information, and producers' names and addresses for software and audiovisual.

Each of the three categories of access points is described further in the following sections.

Subject Focus Fields

Search by the keyword in title, abstract or full text fields when the topic is so specific or so new there is no appropriate CINAHL subject heading, or when the CINAHL subject heading was added recently and older material is needed.

It is important to remember that all words in the title, title clarification, and abstract are searchable.

Cinahl indexers sometimes clarify the title (title clarification) when the title of the work is vague. Title clarification helps you to judge the value of the material indexed. The clarification is preceded by ellipses (...). Both American and British spellings may be present and must be accounted for when searching.

For information about additional subject focus fields please see Appendix 5.

Bibliographic Fields

Search for an author's name when you know that a person has written articles on your topic.

In the CINAHL® database you can search for both personal and corporate authors.

The personal author format is the last name followed by one or more initials. Full first or middle names are never used. Up to three initials are entered as they appear in the article. If an individual uses more than one form of the name, more than one form will appear in the index. For example, Virginia Saba could be searched as Saba V or Saba VK. For journal articles all authors and/or corporate authors are listed.

For information about additional bibliographic fields, please see Appendix 5.

Fields with Additional Information

Search to locate books, journals, educational software, audiovisuals, dissertations, or pamphlets.

The names and addresses of producers and/or distributors of software and audiovisuals are cited in full. Example: Milner-Fenwick, 2125 Greenspring Drive, Timonium MD 21093, phone: 800-432-8433.

Book records include the publisher and place of publication. Example: Sage Publ (Thousand Oaks, CA) ** 1996 (264 p).

For fields with additional information please see Appendix 5.

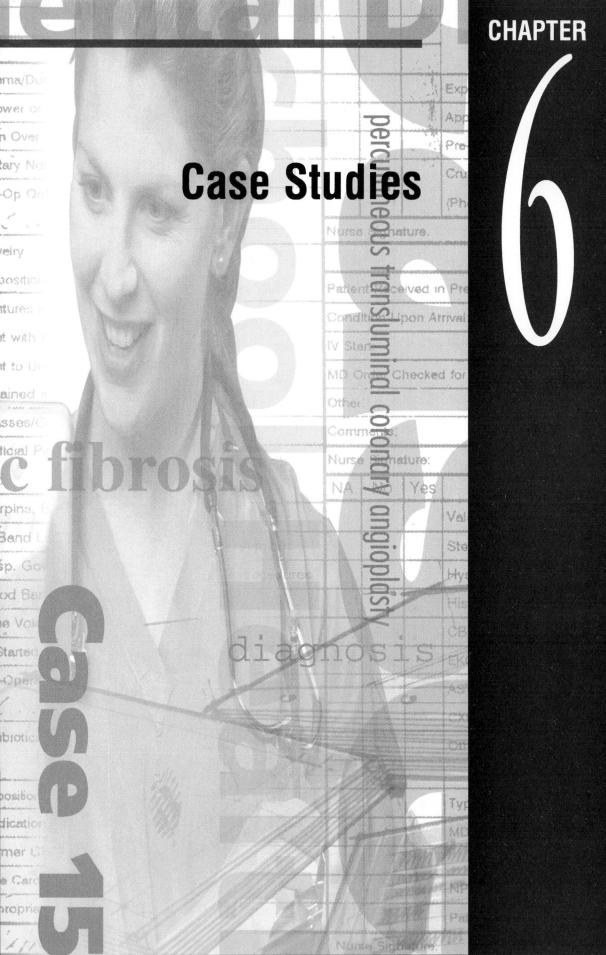

Case Studies

he following 24 case studies were designed to give you an opportunity to practice searching the literature using actual examples from nursing practice. To determine the content of the case studies, four primary concept areas were chosen. Specific topics were then further defined under each primary concept area as follows:

1 Client-Centered Concepts
Culture and Ethnicity
Growth and Development
Chronicity
High-Risk Populations
Family and Support Networks
Access to Resources
Client Education
Health Promotion

2 Nurse-Centered Concepts and Roles
Case Management
Managed Care
Quality Management
Leadership and Management
Ethics
Research
Nursing Informatics
Advocacy

3 Nursing Care Delivery Settings
Hospital
Ambulatory Care
Home
School
Community
Long Term Care

4 Clinical Specialties
Perinatal
Pediatrics
Medical
Surgical
Psychiatric/Mental Health
Gerontology

The case studies were then developed to include two or more of these content areas. Use the case study matrix on the next page to choose the case studies that are of most interest to you.

Read the case study and go to a CINAHL® database computer search station. At the conclusion of the case study is a search formulation strategy that has been developed using the Six Step Process. Sign on to the CINAHL database and conduct the search as it is outlined in the Six Step Process.* Discover what citations on the topic are available. After one or two "practice" case studies, make your own search strategy and compare it against the strategy in the manual. Or use the search

Information RN Case Study Concept Matrix

CLIENT-CENTERED CONCEPTS

Topic	Case Study
Culture and Ethnicity	4,11,15
Growth and Development	1,7,13,20
Chronicity	2,16,23
High-Risk Populations	3,6,10,12,13,17,20
Family and Support Networks	1,14,18
Access to Resources	3,6,7,10
Client Education	3,4,8,14,18
Health Promotion	3,4,7,20,24

NURSE-CENTERED CONCEPTS AND ROLES

Topic	Case Study
Case Management	3,4,6,14
Managed Care	9,10,21
Quality Management	2,5,10
Leadership and Management	5,13,19
Ethics	1,10,16
Research	7,12
Nursing Informatics	12
Advocacy	1,2,11,16,17,20

NURSING CARE DELIVERY SETTINGS

Topic	Case Study
Hospital	1,5,8,9,10,15,19,21
Ambulatory Care	11,12,14
Home	3,4,18,22,23
School	7,20
Community	6,13,17,22,24
Long Term Care	2,16

CLINICAL SPECIALTIES

Topic	Case Study
Perinatal	3,15,17,19
Pediatrics	1,7,8,13
Medical	4,10,12,13,18
Surgical	5,11
Psychiatric/Mental Health	6,14,20,23
Gerontology	2,16,23

strategy principles to search other electronic databases to see what you can uncover. By practicing the art of searching the literature using these case studies, you will be developing expertise in finding information about nursing and health care. With this information, you can continue to expand your knowledge to achieve excellence in nursing practice in an ever-changing health care environment.

As there are several ways of accessing the CINAHL database (World Wide Web, CD-ROM, various online vendors, etc.) specific instructions for signing on and using a particular interface are not included in this guide. Ask your librarian for instruction on signing on and using the CINAHL database.

CASE STUDY 1

Joshua is a 16-year-old male who was diagnosed with chronic myelogenous leukemia (CML) one year ago. His most recent hospitalization began three months ago to undergo a series of chemotherapy and total body irradiation in preparation for bone marrow transplantation (BMT). Since the BMT, Joshua developed graft versus host disease and his condition has progressed downward during the last month. Currently he is losing 5-6 liters of watery, bloody stool a day as his GI tract continues to slough off. Joshua is NPO and receiving TPN. Yesterday's blood values were: Hgb: 6.4, Hct: 18.1, WBC: 800, Platelets: 16,000. As a result of these blood values, Joshua is receiving round-the-clock blood products. His BUN is 113 and creatinine is 2.6, indicating a threat of kidney failure. A total bilirubin value of 27 indicates liver failure. His skin shows petechiae, rash, sloughing, jaundice, and pruritus. Joshua's medication list includes: ceftazidime 2 gm IV q 8 °, clindamycin, 300 mg IV q 8 °, fluconazole 100 mg IV qd, ganciclovir 375 mg IV qd, Septra 10 cc IV bid, vancomycin 900 mg IV q 36 °, prednisone 70 mg IV q 12 °, $NaHCO_3$ 70 meq q6 °, Benadryl 25-50 mg IV q4 ° PRN, and Dilantin 300 mg IV q 12 °.

Joshua has mentioned to you that he is ready to "go home," suggesting he is accepting the inevitability of his death, yet he has posted a colorful sign on his door which reads, "If you don't think I'm going to make it, don't come in!" He has started talking about all the things in life he has never done (like graduate from high school and have sex), but he also is able to talk about his accomplishments. He is alternately demanding, belligerent, and hostile, and appreciative, compliant, and reflective. He has confided in you that he is tired of fighting and wonders whether there is any point to continuing all the medications.

His mother and current stepfather (his mother has been married 4 times) have been living in a nearby motel throughout this hospitalization because they live in another state, and are at the hospital every day. The mother, who is the only person who can legally make decisions regarding Joshua's treatment, refuses to acknowledge the hopelessness of Joshua's condition. Her refusal to terminate treatment in spite of the hopeless prognosis offered by Joshua's doctors has led to a hospital ethics committee review of the case.

As the nurse assigned to work with Joshua and his family, you are faced with many challenges. First, for an understanding of the developmental needs of a maturing adolescent you search the literature using the term *Adolescent Development*.

To increase your understanding of how you can help Joshua accept his death you then do the following literature search using the six step process:

1 Plan your search strategy ahead of time

2 Break down your search topic into components

You wish to increase your understanding of how you can help Joshua accept his death. Decide on the keywords, synonyms, or related terms of your search. The diagram below shows terms you should have considered. They have been grouped to make the searching process easier.

What are the keywords, synonyms, or related terms?

- death education • death counseling • counseling • death
- attitude to death • death • coping
- terminal care

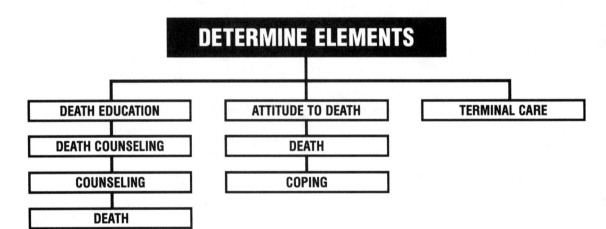

3 Check for subject headings in the Subject Heading List of the CINAHL® database

The following chart displays the subject headings exactly as they appear in the CINAHL Thesaurus.

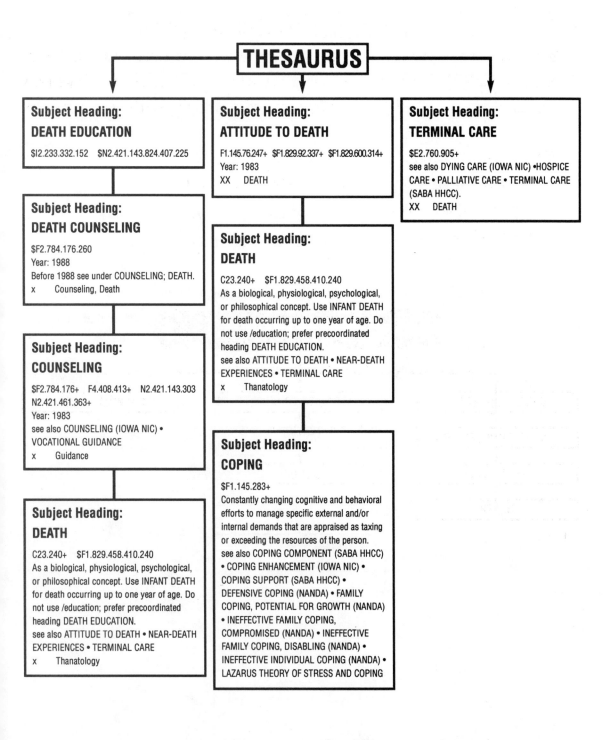

THESAURUS

Subject Heading:
DEATH EDUCATION

$I2.233.332.152 $N2.421.143.824.407.225

Subject Heading:
DEATH COUNSELING

$F2.784.176.260
Year: 1988
Before 1988 see under COUNSELING; DEATH.
x   Counseling, Death

Subject Heading:
COUNSELING

$F2.784.176+   F4.408.413+   N2.421.143.303
N2.421.461.363+
Year: 1983
see also COUNSELING (IOWA NIC) •
VOCATIONAL GUIDANCE
x   Guidance

Subject Heading:
DEATH

C23.240+ $F1.829.458.410.240
As a biological, physiological, psychological, or philosophical concept. Use INFANT DEATH for death occurring up to one year of age. Do not use /education; prefer precoordinated heading DEATH EDUCATION.
see also ATTITUDE TO DEATH • NEAR-DEATH EXPERIENCES • TERMINAL CARE
x   Thanatology

Subject Heading:
ATTITUDE TO DEATH

F1.145.76.247+ $F1.829.92.337+ $F1.829.600.314+
Year: 1983
XX   DEATH

Subject Heading:
DEATH

C23.240+ $F1.829.458.410.240
As a biological, physiological, psychological, or philosophical concept. Use INFANT DEATH for death occurring up to one year of age. Do not use /education; prefer precoordinated heading DEATH EDUCATION.
see also ATTITUDE TO DEATH • NEAR-DEATH EXPERIENCES • TERMINAL CARE
x   Thanatology

Subject Heading:
COPING

$F1.145.283+
Constantly changing cognitive and behavioral efforts to manage specific external and/or internal demands that are appraised as taxing or exceeding the resources of the person.
see also COPING COMPONENT (SABA HHCC) • COPING ENHANCEMENT (IOWA NIC) • COPING SUPPORT (SABA HHCC) • DEFENSIVE COPING (NANDA) • FAMILY COPING, POTENTIAL FOR GROWTH (NANDA) • INEFFECTIVE FAMILY COPING, COMPROMISED (NANDA) • INEFFECTIVE FAMILY COPING, DISABLING (NANDA) • INEFFECTIVE INDIVIDUAL COPING (NANDA) • LAZARUS THEORY OF STRESS AND COPING

Subject Heading:
TERMINAL CARE

$E2.760.905+
see also DYING CARE (IOWA NIC) •HOSPICE CARE • PALLIATIVE CARE • TERMINAL CARE (SABA HHCC).
XX   DEATH

4 Decide which operators and limits you need

A OPERATORS

- Use operator "OR" to connect synonymous or related terms – for example, *Death Education* OR *Death Counseling*.
- Use operator "AND" to connect the different components – for example, *Death* AND *Coping*.

B LIMITS

- Joshua is an adolescent, so limit your search using the population group *adolescence*.

C CONDUCTING YOUR SEARCHES

- You will be conducting your search using separate components and then combining these components to obtain the actual list of materials on your topic.

1 The first group of terms you will search for will be *Death Education – Death Counseling*. In this search you wish to include earlier material – the history note for the subject heading *Death Counseling* tells you to search *Counseling* and *Death* for material before 1988.

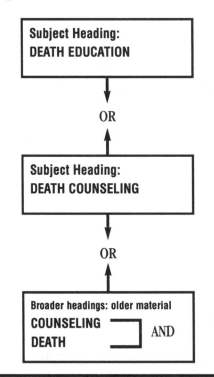

2 The second group of terms you will search for will be *Attitude to Death –
Death* "AND" *Coping*.

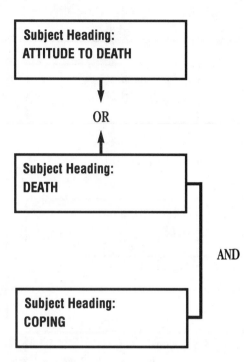

3 *Terminal Care* will then be searched.

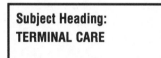

4 Finally, combine the three components and limit by *adolescence*.

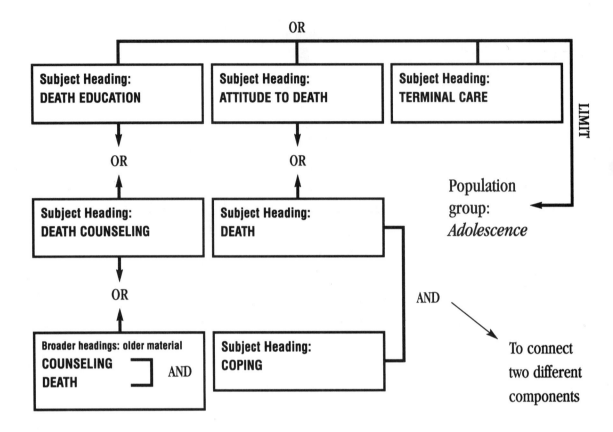

5   Run your search

6   View the results

NOTES

CASE STUDY 2

Mr. Jackson is a 72-year-old man who has just been admitted to the skilled nursing facility (SNF) where you have been hired as a new nurse. Mr. Jackson's medical history includes an acute myocardial infarction (AMI) four years ago and a cerebral vascular accident (CVA) six months ago which left him with left-sided weakness. Since the stroke he has learned to use a walker for exercise, but requires assistance with ambulation to ensure he does not fall. Three weeks ago Mr. Jackson's wife of 48 years died suddenly from a heart attack. In addition to doing all his cooking and cleaning, she had been an active participant in his rehabilitation, assisting him with bathing, dressing, and ambulation. Since her death Mr. Jackson has had no one to take care of him. His three children, who all live on the opposite coast, decided the only solution was to place him in a nursing home.

During your initial meeting with Mr. Jackson, you find that he is pleasant and eager for conversation. He enjoys reminiscing about his wife and takes great pride in the accomplishments of all his children. You find out that he had been a postal worker before he retired and enjoys playing cards, watching game shows on TV, and reading mystery novels. His health status is good, although his daily medications include Inderal 120 mg bid and Coumadin 5 mg qd. You assess that he requires assistance with bathing, getting dressed, and ambulating, but is able to groom himself and eat without assistance. Although he hated having to leave his own home, he recognizes that living in a nursing home was the only option for him after his wife died. He states that he is eager to meet the other residents and make new friends. He asks if there are any other residents who like to play pinochle.

During the next four weeks you notice that Mr. Jackson rapidly deteriorates. He no longer greets you in the morning and practically has to be forced to get out of bed. He has become incontinent of urine and is increasingly emotionally withdrawn. You notice that every day he participates less and less in his activities of daily living. Today you even had to shave him because he refused to do it himself. You have also noticed that he rarely ambulates with his walker and have seen other nurses put him in a wheelchair to get him to the dining room. He now spends most days alone in his room slumped over in his chair.

1 Plan your search strategy ahead of time

2 Break down your search topic into components

You are concerned about Mr. Jackson's rapid deterioration and suspect he is suffering from depression. You want to facilitate a more positive adjustment to the nursing home environment. You want to learn more about depression in the elderly and you hope to gain knowledge of how nurses can increase the quality of life in nursing home residents. Decide on the keywords, synonyms, or related terms of your search. The diagram below shows the terms you should have considered. They have been grouped to make the searching process easier.

What are the keywords, synonyms, or related terms?

- depression • loneliness • personal loss • bereavement • quality of life
- long term care • nursing home patients

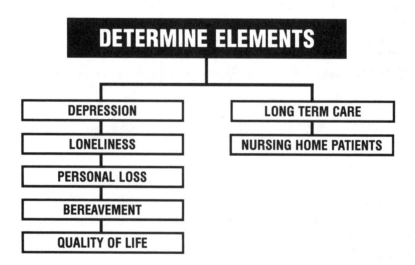

3 Check for subject headings in the Subject Heading List of the CINAHL® database

The following chart displays the subject headings exactly as they appear in the CINAHL Thesaurus.

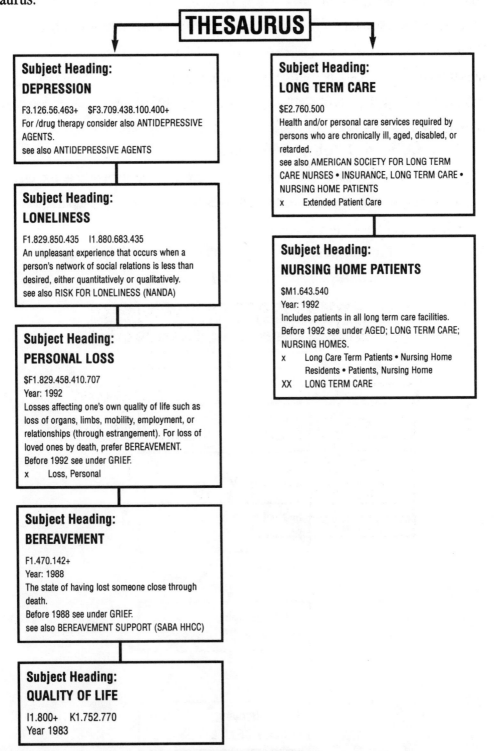

THESAURUS

Subject Heading:
DEPRESSION

F3.126.56.463+ $F3.709.438.100.400+
For /drug therapy consider also ANTIDEPRESSIVE
AGENTS.
see also ANTIDEPRESSIVE AGENTS

Subject Heading:
LONELINESS

F1.829.850.435   I1.880.683.435
An unpleasant experience that occurs when a
person's network of social relations is less than
desired, either quantitatively or qualitatively.
see also RISK FOR LONELINESS (NANDA)

Subject Heading:
PERSONAL LOSS

$F1.829.458.410.707
Year: 1992
Losses affecting one's own quality of life such as
loss of organs, limbs, mobility, employment, or
relationships (through estrangement). For loss of
loved ones by death, prefer BEREAVEMENT.
Before 1992 see under GRIEF.
x   Loss, Personal

Subject Heading:
BEREAVEMENT

F1.470.142+
Year: 1988
The state of having lost someone close through
death.
Before 1988 see under GRIEF.
see also BEREAVEMENT SUPPORT (SABA HHCC)

Subject Heading:
QUALITY OF LIFE

I1.800+   K1.752.770
Year 1983

Subject Heading:
LONG TERM CARE

$E2.760.500
Health and/or personal care services required by
persons who are chronically ill, aged, disabled, or
retarded.
see also AMERICAN SOCIETY FOR LONG TERM
CARE NURSES • INSURANCE, LONG TERM CARE •
NURSING HOME PATIENTS
x   Extended Patient Care

Subject Heading:
NURSING HOME PATIENTS

$M1.643.540
Year: 1992
Includes patients in all long term care facilities.
Before 1992 see under AGED; LONG TERM CARE;
NURSING HOMES.
x   Long Care Term Patients • Nursing Home
        Residents • Patients, Nursing Home
XX   LONG TERM CARE

4 Decide which operators and limits you need

A OPERATORS

- Use operator "OR" to connect synonymous or related terms – for example, *Depression* OR *Loneliness.*

- Use operator "AND" to connect the different components.

B LIMITS

- Mr. Jackson is 72 years old, so limit your search using the population group *aged.*

C CONDUCTING YOUR SEARCHES

- You will be conducting your search using separate components and then combining these components to obtain the actual list of materials on your topic.

  1 The first group of terms you will search for will be *Depression – Loneliness – Personal Loss – Bereavement – Quality of Life.*

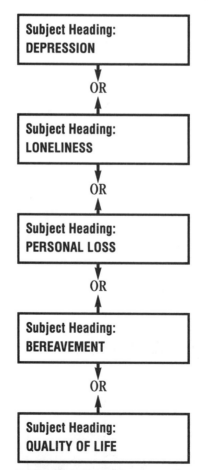

2 The second group of terms you will search for is *Long Term Care – Nursing Home Patients*.

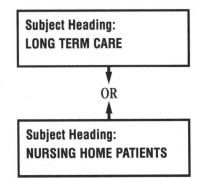

3 Finally, combine the components using the operator "AND", and limit your search to *aged*.

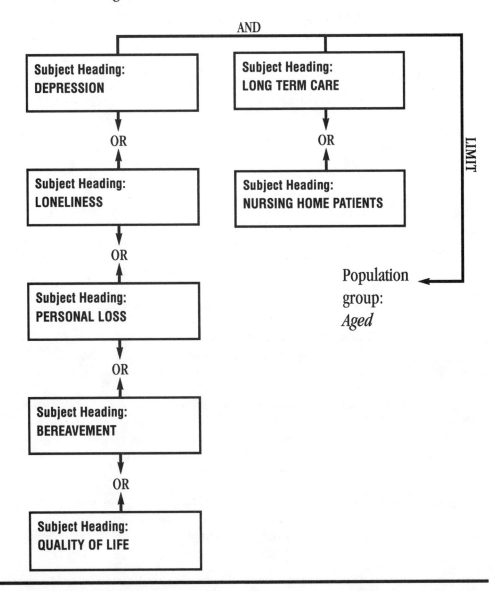

5   Run your search

6   View the results

NOTES

CASE STUDY 3

Tisha is a 15-year-old girl who came to the public health clinic for a pregnancy test, which was positive. Following a history and exam it was estimated that she is 3 1/2 months along in the pregnancy. You are a nursing student and have been assigned to be the public health nurse who will follow Tisha with home visits throughout her pregnancy. During your first visit you assess her general health, living situation, and learning needs.

You discover that Tisha lives with her mother, who is an active alcoholic, and her 17-year-old sister, who is addicted to cocaine. Her older sister has had three children who have all been taken from her by Child Protective Services. Tisha reports having dropped out of school about the same time she became pregnant. She admits to drinking (but only on the weekends) and to smoking pot. She says she refuses to use cocaine because she saw what it did to her sister. She also smokes about half a pack of cigarettes a day. Her biggest concern about her pregnancy right now is that she doesn't want to look fat, because then her boyfriend won't want to make love to her. She says that she rarely eats breakfast, and has never liked milk or vegetables.

Tisha is excited about the thought of having a baby because "they're so cute." She thinks she will be a good mother because "I'm going to give this baby more love than my mother ever gave me." Tisha does not know who the father of her baby is, because she had unprotected sex with three different boys during the time when she would have gotten pregnant. Tisha's mother is not happy about her daughter having a baby so young, but states she believes Tisha will be a good mother because she is not on cocaine like her sister.

You recognize that Tisha has many learning needs regarding substance abuse, nutrition and STD prevention. You know from Tisha's age, history of smoking and drinking, and her poor eating habits that this baby is at high risk for multiple health and developmental problems. In addition, Tisha's economic level, family situation and educational history put her at high risk of additional pregnancies while still a teenager.

1 Plan your search strategy ahead of time

2 Break down your search topic into components

You have two weeks before your next visit with Tisha and you decide to search the literature for help in setting realistic goals with your client. Decide on the keywords, synonyms, or related terms of your search. The diagram below shows the terms you should have considered. They have been grouped to make the searching process easier.

What are the keywords, synonyms, or related terms?
- pregnancy in adolescence • pregnancy, high risk
- safe sex • smoking cessation • nutritional counseling • substance abuse, perinatal
- patient education • prenatal care • community health nursing

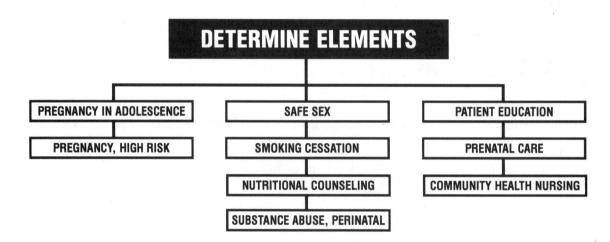

3 Check for subject headings in the Subject Heading List of the CINAHL® database

The following chart displays the subject headings exactly as they appear in the CINAHL Thesaurus.

THESAURUS

Subject Heading:
PREGNANCY IN ADOLESCENCE

G8.520.420.770+ $I1.880.735.640+
Year: 1983
Consider also ADOLESCENT FATHERS;
ADOLESCENT MOTHERS. For pregnancy in
early adolescence or childhood, consider
MATERNAL AGE 14 AND UNDER
x   Adolescent Pregnancy • Teenage
     Pregnancy

Subject Heading:
PREGNANCY, HIGH RISK

$G8.520.769.655
Year: 1989
Consider also specific Pregnancy
Complication Terms.
Before 1989 see under PREGNANCY
COMPLICATIONS; Specific Pregnancy
Complications Terms.
see also PERINATAL NURSING
x   High Risk Pregnancy

Subject Heading:
SAFE SEX

$F1.145.794.850
Year: 1993
Sexual practices designed to prevent the
spread of sexually transmitted diseases.
Before 1993 see under SEXUALITY;
SEXUALLY TRANSMITTED
DISEASES/prevention and control.

Subject Heading:
SMOKING CESSATION

F1.145.466.753.800
Year: 1992
Discontinuing the smoking habit.
Before 1992 see under SMOKING/prevention
and control; SMOKING CESSATION
PROGRAMS.
see also SMOKING CESSATION ASSISTANCE
(IOWA NIC)

Subject Heading:
NUTRITIONAL COUNSELING

$N2.421.543.620
Year: 1993
Before 1993 see under NUTRITION.
see also NUTRITIONAL COUNSELING (IOWA
NIC) • TEACHING: PRESCRIBED DIET (IOWA
NIC)

Subject Heading:
SUBSTANCE ABUSE, PERINATAL

$C13.703.722.815 $F1.145.905.815
$F3.709.597.780.610.815 $F3.709.615.815
$I1.880.735.820.815
Year: 1992
Abuse of any substance, including alcohol, by
the mother before her child's birth and/or
during the breast feeding period.
Searchable electronically since 1983.
see also NEONATAL ABSTINENCE
SYNDROME
x   Perinatal Drug Exposure • Perinatal
     Substance Abuse • Prenatal Drug
     Exposure
XX   INFANT, DRUG-EXPOSED •
     MATERNAL-FETAL EXCHANGE •
     NEONATAL ABSTINENCE SYNDROME

Subject Heading:
PATIENT EDUCATION

I2.233.332.500+ $N2.421.143.824.407.680+
A combination of learning and motivation
activities designed to educate patients and
family members about disease states or
procedures and appropriate methods for self-
care. May occur in either inpatient or
outpatient settings. Coordinate with specific
disease or procedure/education. For articles
that contain examples of patient education
materials search for the document type
"consumer/patient teaching materials."
see also KNOWLEDGE DEFICIT (NANDA) •
TEACHING: DISEASE PROCESS (IOWA NIC) •
TEACHING: GROUP (IOWA NIC) • TEACHING:
INDIVIDUAL (IOWA NIC) • TEACHING:
INFANT CARE (IOWA NIC) • TEACHING:
PRESCRIBED ACTIVITY/EXERCISE (IOWA
NIC) • TEACHING: PRESCRIBED DIET (IOWA
NIC)• TEACHING: PRESCRIBED MEDICATION
(IOWA NIC) • TEACHING: PSYCHOMOTOR
SKILL (IOWA NIC)
x   Education of Patients

Subject Heading:
PRENATAL CARE

$E2.760.525.627.710+ $N2.421.143.620.704+
Care of the mother and fetus from the time of
conception until the onset of labor.
see also CHILDBIRTH EDUCATION •
PERINATAL CARE • PRENATAL CARE (IOWA
NIC)
XX   PREGNANCY

Subject Heading:
COMMUNITY HEALTH NURSING

$G2.478.675.167+   N2.421.143.150+
$N2.421.533.167+
see also HOME NURSING, PROFESSIONAL •
HOME VISITS
x   Community Based Nursing • District
     Nursing • Health Visitors •
     Neighborhood Nursing • Public Health
     Nursing

4 Decide which operators and limits you need

A OPERATORS

- Use operator "OR" to connect synonymous or related terms – for example, *Pregnancy in Adolescence* OR *Pregnancy, High Risk*.
- Use operator "AND" to connect the different components.

B LIMITS

- This case study involves a 15-year-old who is pregnant, so limit your search by population groups using *female, pregnancy,* and *adolescence.*

C CONDUCTING YOUR SEARCHES

- You will be conducting your search using separate components and then combining these components to obtain the actual list of materials on your topic.

  1 The first group of terms you will search for will be *Pregnancy in Adolescence – Pregnancy, High Risk.*

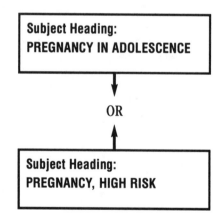

2 The second group of terms you will search for will be *Safe Sex – Smoking Cessation – Nutritional Counseling – Substance Abuse, Perinatal.*

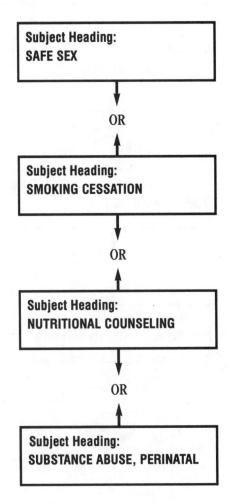

3   The third group of terms you will search for will be *Patient Education –
Prenatal Care – Community Health Nursing.*

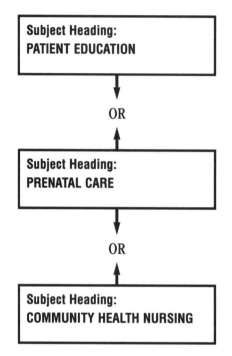

4 Put the three pieces together using the operators: [*Pregnancy in Adolescence* OR *Pregnancy, High Risk* OR *Safe Sex* OR *Smoking Cessation* OR *Nutritional Counseling* OR *Substance Abuse, Perinatal*] AND [*Patient Education* OR *Prenatal Care* OR *Community Health Nursing*] and limit your search to *pregnancy, female, and adolescence*.

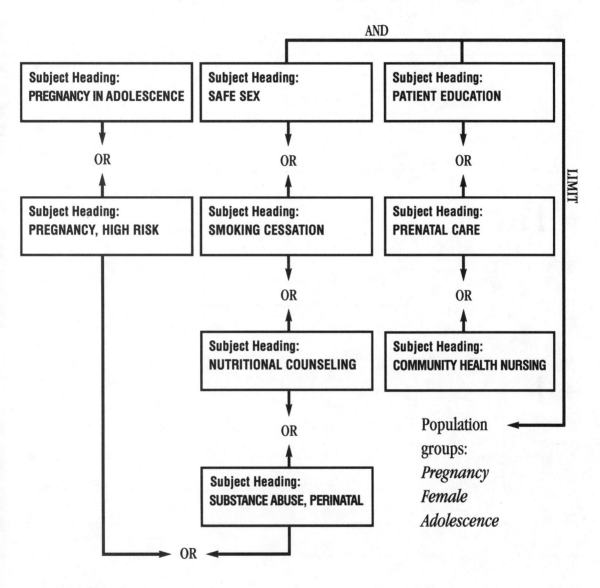

5 Run your search

6 View the results

NOTES

CASE STUDY 4

Ms. Carter is a 34-year-old African-American woman who has just been diagnosed with Type II diabetes and severe hypertension, and you are the community health nurse assigned to provide client education and monitor her at home following her discharge from the hospital. During your assessment just before her discharge you discover the following information.

Ms. Carter is 5'4" tall and weighs 220 lbs. Her vital signs are T-36.9 °, P-86, R-18, and BP-168/100 (on admission it had been 196/112). Except for the usual childhood illnesses and a hernia repair at age 12, she never had any previous medical problems. Her mother and father were both overweight, and both died in their 50's due to hypertension and coronary artery disease.

Ms. Carter reports battling her weight since she was a little girl. These weight loss attempts included fad diets, starvation, self-induced vomiting, use of laxatives and medically supervised liquid diets. Although she was able to lose weight with these different methods, she always gained it back. She reluctantly admits that she attempted suicide at age 26 when her boyfriend left her and she lost her job under circumstances that clearly suggested weight discrimination. After several years in psychotherapy, she says she was finally able to accept herself. She then started her own boutique specializing in fashions for "full-figured" women. She helped start a local "Fat is Beautiful" support group and currently volunteers once a week for the local suicide prevention hotline. Ms. Carter freely admits that she loves to eat, especially salty and fried foods and anything chocolate. She states, however, that trying to be thin almost killed her and that it wasn't until she accepted herself as a fat person that she learned to be happy.

Besides teaching her how to take her own blood pressure, test her own blood sugar and learn the symptoms of hypo/hyperglycemia you know that a major part of your work will be in nutritional counseling. Because of Ms. Carter's prior failure with weight loss and her struggle to accept herself, you understand that being overweight and being told to follow a strict diet have unique meanings to her. You are cautious about implementing your regular diabetic diet teaching with its rigid calorie demands. At the same time you know that Ms. Carter's health status requires immediate action.

1 Plan your search strategy ahead of time

2 Break down your search topic into components

You decide to search the literature on how to approach your nutritional counseling with Ms. Carter. What are reasonable weight loss and blood pressure goals with which you might expect Ms. Carter to agree? How can you present the need for Ms. Carter to change her diet and lose weight while still affirming her personal worth and valuing her accomplishments as a "fat person"? Decide on the keywords, synonyms, or related terms of your search. The diagram below shows the terms you should have considered. They have been grouped to make the searching process easier.

What are the keywords, synonyms, or related terms?
- diabetes mellitus, non-insulin-dependent • blacks
- diet therapy • weight control
- health education

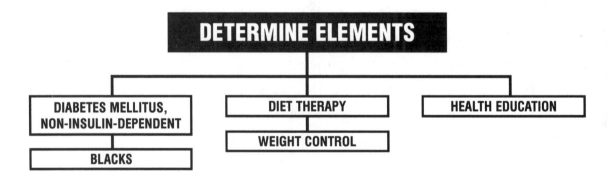

3 Check for subject headings in the Subject Heading List of the CINAHL® database

The following chart displays the subject headings exactly as they appear in the CINAHL Thesaurus.

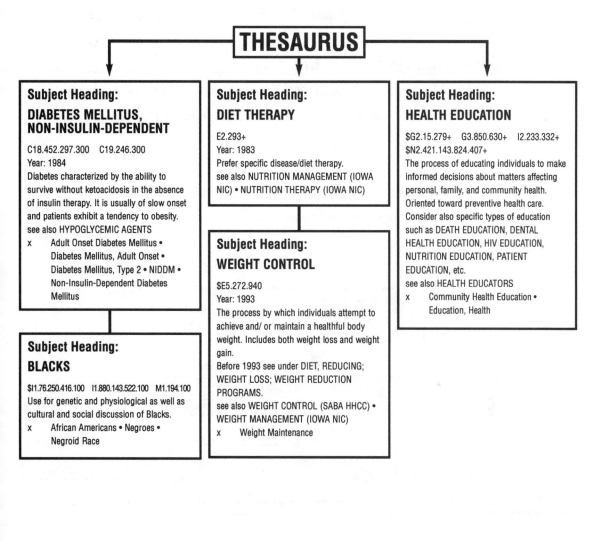

THESAURUS

Subject Heading:
DIABETES MELLITUS, NON-INSULIN-DEPENDENT

C18.452.297.300   C19.246.300
Year: 1984
Diabetes characterized by the ability to survive without ketoacidosis in the absence of insulin therapy. It is usually of slow onset and patients exhibit a tendency to obesity.
see also HYPOGLYCEMIC AGENTS
x   Adult Onset Diabetes Mellitus •
       Diabetes Mellitus, Adult Onset •
       Diabetes Mellitus, Type 2 • NIDDM •
       Non-Insulin-Dependent Diabetes
       Mellitus

Subject Heading:
BLACKS

$I1.76.250.416.100   I1.880.143.522.100   M1.194.100
Use for genetic and physiological as well as cultural and social discussion of Blacks.
x   African Americans • Negroes •
       Negroid Race

Subject Heading:
DIET THERAPY

E2.293+
Year: 1983
Prefer specific disease/diet therapy.
see also NUTRITION MANAGEMENT (IOWA NIC) • NUTRITION THERAPY (IOWA NIC)

Subject Heading:
WEIGHT CONTROL

$E5.272.940
Year: 1993
The process by which individuals attempt to achieve and/ or maintain a healthful body weight. Includes both weight loss and weight gain.
Before 1993 see under DIET, REDUCING; WEIGHT LOSS; WEIGHT REDUCTION PROGRAMS.
see also WEIGHT CONTROL (SABA HHCC) • WEIGHT MANAGEMENT (IOWA NIC)
x   Weight Maintenance

Subject Heading:
HEALTH EDUCATION

$G2.15.279+   G3.850.630+   I2.233.332+
$N2.421.143.824.407+
The process of educating individuals to make informed decisions about matters affecting personal, family, and community health. Oriented toward preventive health care. Consider also specific types of education such as DEATH EDUCATION, DENTAL HEALTH EDUCATION, HIV EDUCATION, NUTRITION EDUCATION, PATIENT EDUCATION, etc.
see also HEALTH EDUCATORS
x   Community Health Education •
       Education, Health

4 Decide which operators you need

A OPERATORS

- Use operator "OR" to connect synonymous or related terms – for example, *Diabetes Mellitus, Non-Insulin-Dependent* OR *Blacks*.

- Use operator "AND" to connect the different components.

B CONDUCTING YOUR SEARCHES

- You will be conducting your search using separate components and then combining these components to obtain the actual list of materials on your topic.

  1 The first group of terms you will search for will be *Diabetes Mellitus, Non-Insulin-Dependent – Blacks*.

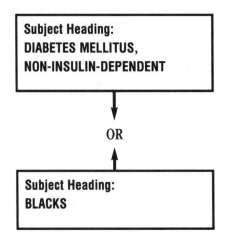

2 The second group of terms you will search for will be *Diet Therapy –
Weight Control.*

When you search *Diet Therapy,* select it and all the specific terms under it
by choosing the "explode" option. This will retrieve all documents on the
broad heading and the more specific headings as well.

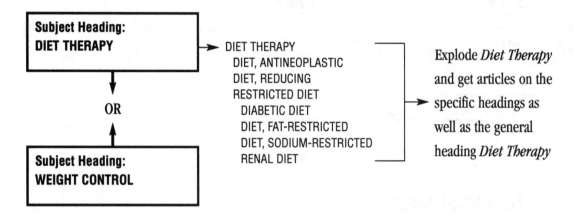

3 Then search for *Health Education*. Choose the "explode" option here as
well.

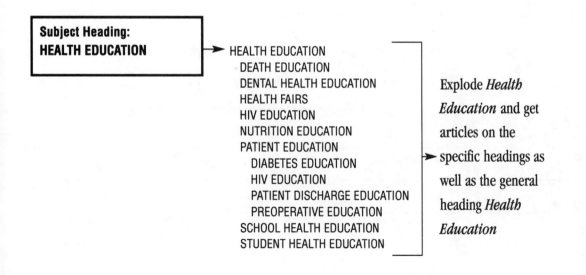

4 Finally, combine the three components with the operator "AND".

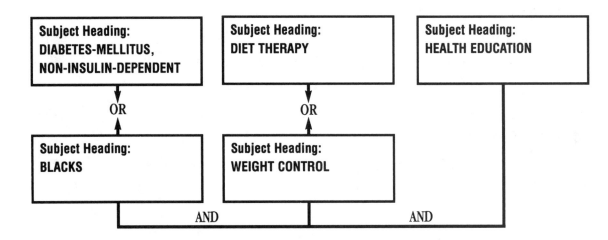

5 Run your search

6 View the results

NOTES

CASE STUDY 5

You are the nurse manger on a 24-bed surgical floor in a 385-bed hospital. You have worked at this hospital for 20 years and have seen many changes in nursing practice and staffing patterns over the years. Ten years ago you remember that primary nursing allowed RNs to take complete care of three or four patients. On your 24-bed unit there would typically have been five to seven RNs, depending on the census and acuity level of the patients. With the change to team nursing, RNs typically are responsible for six to eight patients and are helped by a Certified Nursing Assistant. At full census, your staffing guidelines are to have three RNs and three CNAs to care for the 24 patients.

Your hospital is undergoing "restructuring" in an effort to be more cost efficient. You have been ordered to cut nursing costs by 10%. You know that your options are to require nursing staff to care for more patients, and/or to adjust the staffing mix to include RNs, LVNs and CNAs. By using more LVNs and CNAs, you know that the RN job description will change to include doing only those tasks that can be legally performed by RNs.

You worry that this will result in more fragmentation of patient care and a feeling among RNs that they are providing assembly line care (e.g., they would end up hanging the IV medications for all the patients on the unit, but would never really get to know any of the patients individually since the LVNs and CNAs would be providing all the rest of the hands-on care).

1 Plan your search strategy ahead of time

2 Break down your search topic into components

You decide to search the literature to get different perspectives on the changing roles of different licensed staff. You want to know what nurses themselves are saying about staffing pattern changes and the resulting changes in their responsibilities and relationships with patients. You want to find out what has worked and what has not worked at other hospitals. Although the financial realities in your institution require that you implement these staffing changes, you hope to find guidelines so the new job descriptions you will write will still ensure patient safety and give nurses job satisfaction. Decide on the keywords, synonyms, or related terms of your search. The diagram below shows terms you should have considered. They have been grouped to make the searching process easier.

What are the keywords, synonyms, or related terms?
- nursing staff, hospital
- differentiated nursing practice • personnel staffing and scheduling
- nurse-patient relations • job satisfaction • nursing outcomes

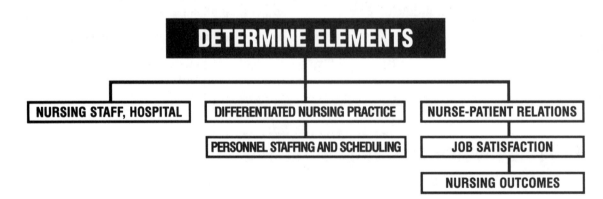

3 Check for subject headings in the Subject Heading List of the CINAHL® database

The following chart displays the subject headings exactly as they appear in the CINAHL Thesaurus.

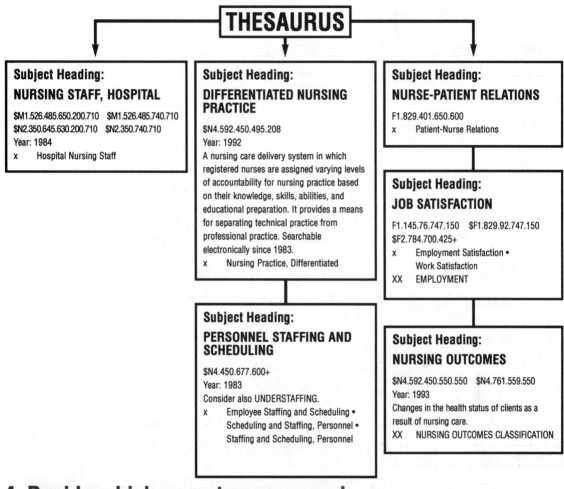

THESAURUS

Subject Heading:
NURSING STAFF, HOSPITAL

$M1.526.485.650.200.710 $M1.526.485.740.710
$N2.350.645.630.200.710 $N2.350.740.710
Year: 1984
x   Hospital Nursing Staff

Subject Heading:
DIFFERENTIATED NURSING PRACTICE

$N4.592.450.495.208
Year: 1992
A nursing care delivery system in which registered nurses are assigned varying levels of accountability for nursing practice based on their knowledge, skills, abilities, and educational preparation. It provides a means for separating technical practice from professional practice. Searchable electronically since 1983.
x   Nursing Practice, Differentiated

Subject Heading:
NURSE-PATIENT RELATIONS

F1.829.401.650.600
x   Patient-Nurse Relations

Subject Heading:
JOB SATISFACTION

F1.145.76.747.150 $F1.829.92.747.150
$F2.784.700.425+
x   Employment Satisfaction •
       Work Satisfaction
XX   EMPLOYMENT

Subject Heading:
PERSONNEL STAFFING AND SCHEDULING

$N4.450.677.600+
Year: 1983
Consider also UNDERSTAFFING.
x   Employee Staffing and Scheduling •
       Scheduling and Staffing, Personnel •
       Staffing and Scheduling, Personnel

Subject Heading:
NURSING OUTCOMES

$N4.592.450.550.550 $N4.761.559.550
Year: 1993
Changes in the health status of clients as a result of nursing care.
XX   NURSING OUTCOMES CLASSIFICATION

4 Decide which operators you need

A OPERATORS

- Use operator "OR" to connect synonymous or related terms – for example, *Differentiated Nursing Practice* OR *Personnel Staffing and Scheduling*.
- Use operator "AND" to connect the different components.

B CONDUCTING YOUR SEARCHES

- You will be conducting your search using separate components and then combining these components to obtain the actual list of materials on your topic.

1 First search for *Nursing Staff, Hospital*.

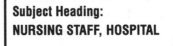

> **Subject Heading:**
> **NURSING STAFF, HOSPITAL**

2 The group of terms you will search for next are *Differentiated Nursing Practice – Personnel Staffing and Scheduling*.

When you search *Personnel Staffing and Scheduling,* select it and all the specific terms under it by choosing the "explode" option.

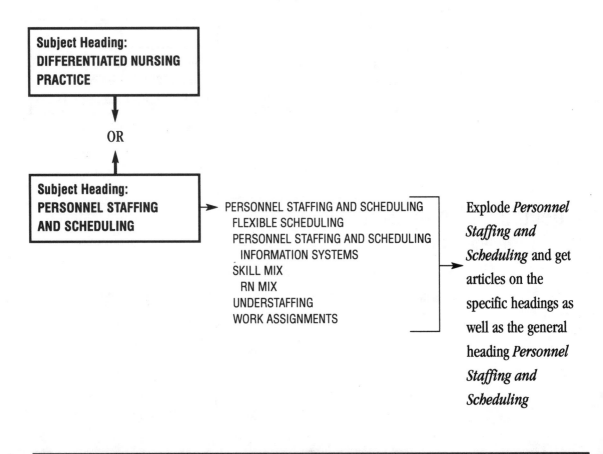

3 The third group of terms you will search for are *Nurse-Patient Relations – Job Satisfaction – Nursing Outcomes*.

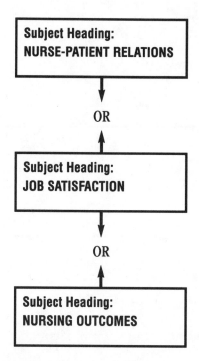

4 Finally, combine the three components with the operator "AND".

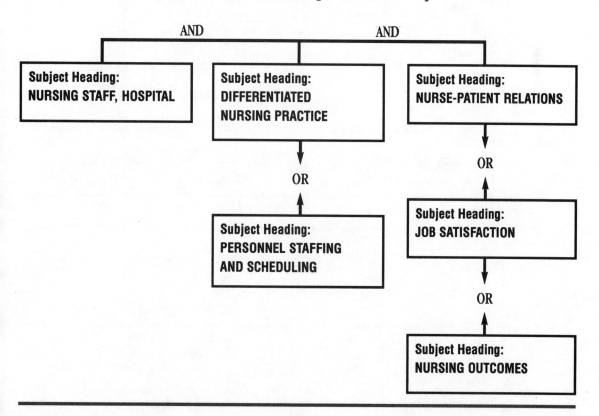

5   Run your search

6   View the results

NOTES

CASE STUDY 6

You are a nursing student doing your community/public health rotation. You are working out of the county public health department making home visits to clients who have been classified as being "non-compliant." You have been assigned to work with Robert, a 45-year-old man who had a cerebral vascular accident (CVA) one year ago related to heavy cocaine use. As a result of the stroke, Robert has left-sided weakness. He can walk short distances only with the help of a cane, has no strength in his left hand and has slurred speech. He is currently living in a subsidized housing project, but prior to his stroke had been homeless for 10 years. In addition, he has a long history of schizophrenia and alcoholism. He also has AIDS.

During your first visit you try to establish rapport with Robert and set mutually acceptable goals. You explain to him that you know he has been seeing doctors at several different drop-in clinics around the city. You understand that these doctors have prescribed different medications for his various medical and psychiatric conditions, not knowing that other medications had already been prescribed. In fact, during a review of the medications which he shows you, you notice that he has three full bottles of Cogentin prescribed by three different doctors. Robert asks you if you can help him get a refill on his inhalers since he has already used up all his Medicaid stickers for prescriptions for this month. You explain to Robert that you can help coordinate the care he is getting from the different providers and manage his medications so he doesn't run out of some meds while having duplicate prescriptions of others. You also suggest that you can work with him to access other services he might need. Initially Robert agrees with this plan.

During the next three months you visit him every week. You set him up with a Medi-set® kit to help him take his meds as prescribed, and contact all the prescribing physicians to inform them of Robert's pattern of using multiple providers. You also help Robert get emergency food at the end of the month since he has run out, and investigate getting a home aid who can help Robert with cleaning his apartment. During your home visits you notice that some days Robert's speech is clear and thought pattern coherent and other days it is almost impossible to understand his words or follow his thought pattern. You know that his stroke, schizophrenia and irregular use of psychotropic medications contribute to this, but you also suspect continuing drug and alcohol use. Even though Robert has denied drinking or using drugs, you know strict housing agency policies regarding any substance use may be preventing him from being honest with you. You also wonder whether AIDS dementia might be playing a part in his changing mental status. You are confused about how to evaluate Robert's condition.

1 Plan your search strategy ahead of time

2 Break down your search topic into components

You decide to search the literature. You are looking for more information about the signs of AIDS dementia and how it can be differentiated from other mental illnesses. You also need to brush up on how different street drugs and alcohol can affect mental status. You are also interested in finding narrative reports of other nurses who have worked with people who have the compound problems of mental illness, substance abuse, and AIDS. You hope that you can gain insight into managing the health needs of a very difficult client. Decide on the keywords, synonyms, or related terms of your search. The diagram below shows terms you should have considered. They have been grouped to make the searching process easier.

What are the keywords, synonyms, or related terms?
- AIDS dementia complex + diagnosis
- mental disorders • acquired immunodeficiency syndrome

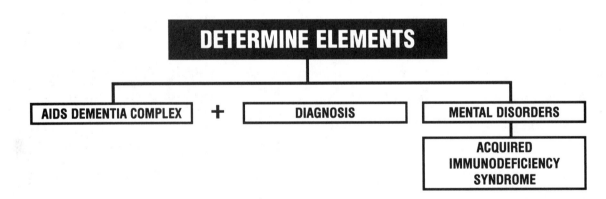

3 Check for subject headings in the Subject Heading List of the CINAHL® database

The following chart displays the subject headings exactly as they appear in the CINAHL Thesaurus.

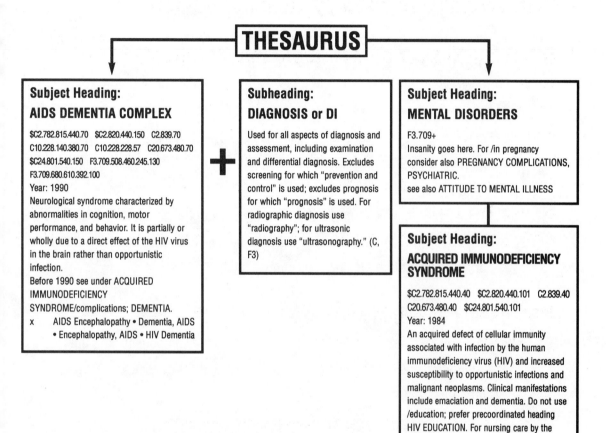

THESAURUS

Subject Heading:

AIDS DEMENTIA COMPLEX

$C2.782.815.440.70 $C2.820.440.150   C2.839.70
C10.228.140.380.70   C10.228.228.57   C20.673.480.70
$C24.801.540.150   F3.709.508.460.245.130
F3.709.680.610.392.100
Year: 1990
Neurological syndrome characterized by abnormalities in cognition, motor performance, and behavior. It is partially or wholly due to a direct effect of the HIV virus in the brain rather than opportunistic infection.
Before 1990 see under ACQUIRED IMMUNODEFICIENCY SYNDROME/complications; DEMENTIA.
x   AIDS Encephalopathy • Dementia, AIDS • Encephalopathy, AIDS • HIV Dementia

+

Subheading:

DIAGNOSIS or DI

Used for all aspects of diagnosis and assessment, including examination and differential diagnosis. Excludes screening for which "prevention and control" is used; excludes prognosis for which "prognosis" is used. For radiographic diagnosis use "radiography"; for ultrasonic diagnosis use "ultrasonography." (C, F3)

Subject Heading:

MENTAL DISORDERS

F3.709+
Insanity goes here. For /in pregnancy consider also PREGNANCY COMPLICATIONS, PSYCHIATRIC.
see also ATTITUDE TO MENTAL ILLNESS

Subject Heading:

ACQUIRED IMMUNODEFICIENCY SYNDROME

$C2.782.815.440.40 $C2.820.440.101   C2.839.40
C20.673.480.40 $C24.801.540.101
Year: 1984
An acquired defect of cellular immunity associated with infection by the human immunodeficiency virus (HIV) and increased susceptibility to opportunistic infections and malignant neoplasms. Clinical manifestations include emaciation and dementia. Do not use /education; prefer precoordinated heading HIV EDUCATION. For nursing care by the specialty use /nursing plus HIV-AIDS NURSING. For nursing care by other specialties (i.e., emergency nursing, critical care nursing) use /nursing and coordinate with that nursing specialty. For /transmission consider HUMAN IMMUNODEFICIENCY VIRUS/transmission.
see also AIDS SERODIAGNOSIS • ATTITUDE TO AIDS • LYMPHOMA, AIDS-RELATED
x   AIDS • Immunodeficiency Syndrome, Acquired • Immunologic Deficiency Syndrome, Acquired

4 Decide which operators and limits you need

A OPERATORS

- Use operator "OR" to connect synonymous or related terms. In this example you wish to browse through two sets at the same time, for example, *AIDS Dementia Complex/Diagnosis* OR (*Mental Disorders* AND *Acquired Immunodeficiency Syndrome*), so use the operator "OR" as a shortcut.

- Use operator "AND" to connect the different components – for example *Mental Disorders* AND *Acquired Immunodeficiency Syndrome*.

B LIMITS

- **Subheadings.** Choose the subheading *diagnosis* when searching *AIDS Dementia Complex* to review material covering only the diagnosis of AIDS dementia complex.

- **Major focus.** Choose to modify the subject headings *Mental Disorders* and *Acquired Immunodeficiency Syndrome* by selecting those materials that focus on these two topics (major subject headings).

C CONDUCTING YOUR SEARCHES

- You will be conducting your search using separate components and then combining these components to obtain the actual list of materials on your topic.

  1 The first term you will search for is *AIDS Dementia Complex*. The search will be limited by the selection of the subheading *Diagnosis*.

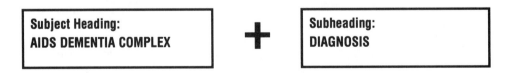

Subject Heading:		Subheading:
AIDS DEMENTIA COMPLEX	**+**	**DIAGNOSIS**

2 The next search will be for *Mental Disorders – Acquired Immunodeficiency Syndrome*. When you search *Mental Disorders* select the broad heading and all the specific terms under it by choosing the "explode" option. Choose material that focuses on the topic for both subject headings by choosing to "restrict to focus" (major subject headings).

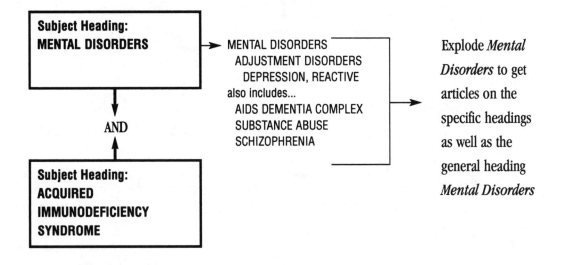

3 Finally, combine the components using the "OR" operator.

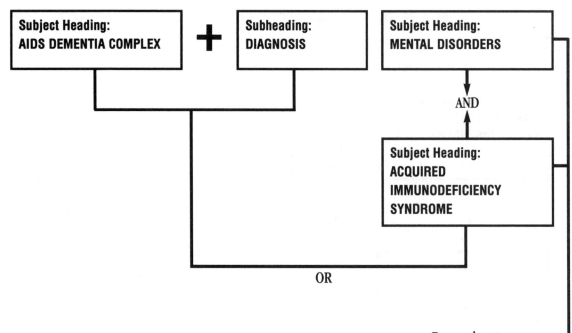

5   Run your search

6   View the results

NOTES

CASE STUDY 7

You are a female school nurse in a large city public high school. Your student health center has been awarded a demonstration grant for a program which combines sex education courses for all grades, comprehensive reproductive services, and referrals. The goal is to reduce the number of teenage pregnancies and sexually transmitted diseases.

Although it was controversial within the community, the program includes free condom distribution with instruction on correct usage. Although program planners initially thought male students would be knocking down the doors to get free condoms, you have noticed that very few have requested them. In fact, a review of the records shows that more female students than male students have requested condoms.

Currently all the staff at the student health center are female. You suspect that more male students would request condoms if they could receive them from a male health worker. Although you are committed to making this program a success, you realize that advocating a change in staffing could mean being replaced by a male nurse. Before you discuss this issue with your supervisor, you decide you need more information.

1 Plan your search strategy ahead of time

2 Break down your search topic into components

In addition to informally talking with boys at school about their comfort level with asking for condoms from the female school nursing staff, you decide to search the literature. You want to know if any research has been done on sexually active adolescent males and their pattern of condom usage. You want to know where they regularly access prophylactics. You know that normal adolescent development includes being shy about discussing sex with the opposite gender. You wonder if there are things you and the other female health workers in your school clinic can do to make accessing condoms more comfortable for male students. You also want to know if other schools with condom distribution programs have encountered this issue and what they have done about it. Decide on the keywords, synonyms, or related terms of your search. The diagram below shows terms you should have considered. They have been grouped to make the searching process easier.

What are the keywords, synonyms, or related terms?

- condoms • contraceptive devices
- sexuality
- school health • school health services

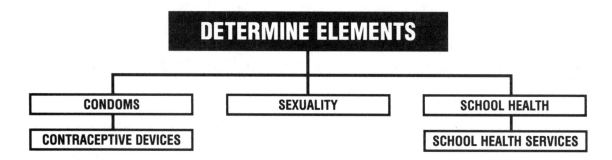

3 Check for subject headings in the Subject Heading List of the CINAHL® database

The following chart displays the subject headings exactly as they appear in the CINAHL Thesaurus.

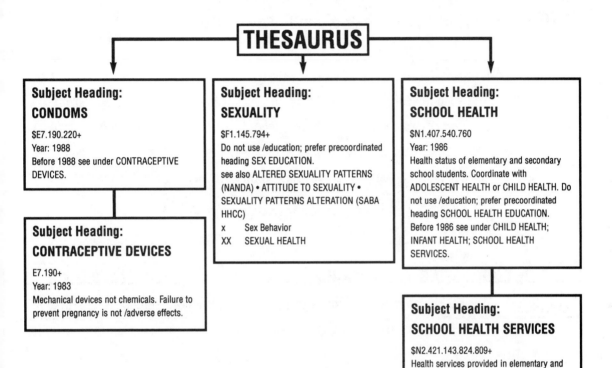

THESAURUS

Subject Heading:
CONDOMS

$E7.190.220+
Year: 1988
Before 1988 see under CONTRACEPTIVE DEVICES.

Subject Heading:
CONTRACEPTIVE DEVICES

E7.190+
Year: 1983
Mechanical devices not chemicals. Failure to prevent pregnancy is not /adverse effects.

Subject Heading:
SEXUALITY

$F1.145.794+
Do not use /education; prefer precoordinated heading SEX EDUCATION.
see also ALTERED SEXUALITY PATTERNS (NANDA) • ATTITUDE TO SEXUALITY • SEXUALITY PATTERNS ALTERATION (SABA HHCC)
x   Sex Behavior
XX   SEXUAL HEALTH

Subject Heading:
SCHOOL HEALTH

$N1.407.540.760
Year: 1986
Health status of elementary and secondary school students. Coordinate with ADOLESCENT HEALTH or CHILD HEALTH. Do not use /education; prefer precoordinated heading SCHOOL HEALTH EDUCATION.
Before 1986 see under CHILD HEALTH; INFANT HEALTH; SCHOOL HEALTH SERVICES.

Subject Heading:
SCHOOL HEALTH SERVICES

$N2.421.143.824.809+
Health services provided in elementary and secondary schools.
see also STUDENT HEALTH SERVICES

4 Decide which operators and limits you need

A OPERATORS

- Use operator "OR" to connect synonymous or related terms – for example, *School Health* OR *School Health Services*.
- Use operator "AND" to connect the different components – for example, (*Condoms* OR *Contraceptive Devices*) AND *Sexuality*.

B LIMITS

- You wish to search for sexuality in adolescence – use the population group limit *adolescence*. The search for (*School Health* OR *School Health Services*) AND (*Condoms* OR *Contraceptive Devices*) does not need to be limited further because the headings *School Health* and *School Health Services* imply the population group.
- Limit the entire search to *male*.

C CONDUCTING YOUR SEARCHES

- You will be conducting your search using separate components and then combining these components to obtain the actual list of material on your topic.

  1 The first group of terms you will search for will be *Condoms – Contraceptive Devices*. In this search you wish to include earlier material. The history note for the subject heading *Condoms* tells you to search *Contraceptive Devices* for material before 1988.

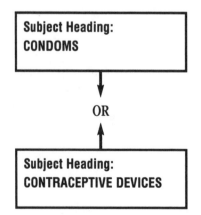

2 The next term you will search for is *Sexuality*. Limit this heading by using the population group *adolescence*.

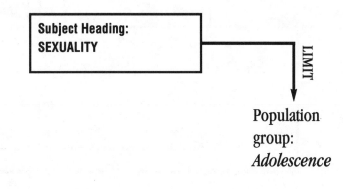

3 The next group of terms you will search for will be *School Health – School Health Services*.

When you search *School Health Services* select the broad heading and all the specific terms under it by choosing the "explode" option.

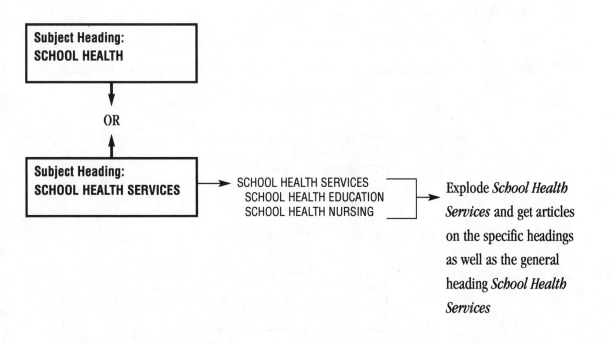

4 Finally, combine the components using the "AND" and "OR" operators.

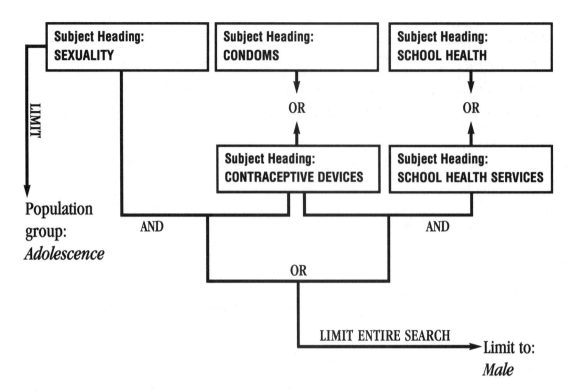

5 Run your search

6 View the results

NOTES

CASE STUDY 8

You are the primary nurse for David, a 7-month-old boy who has been newly diagnosed with cystic fibrosis (CF). David's mother, who is staying with him at the hospital, is a 19-year-old single mother who also has a three year old son and is 2-months pregnant. David presents with the typical symptoms of CF: rhonchi throughout all lung fields which are audible without a stethoscope, pneumonia which is being treated with several different antibiotics, use of accessory muscles for breathing, numerous frothy, foul smelling stools, and being in the 5th percentile in weight for children his age. A chloride sweat test done two days ago confirmed the diagnosis of cystic fibrosis.

After the test results came back and the doctor informed David's mother, you assessed how much she understood of what the doctor had told her. You realized she would need a lot of education, as most parents of CF children do, and so you began by providing her with the standard packet of literature given to parents. This packet included booklets which describe the pathophysiology of CF, give instructions on doing chest physiotherapy, provide information about pancreatic enzymes, and give guidelines to meet the nutritional requirements of children with CF. You explained to David's mother that you understand how overwhelmed she must be with this new diagnosis, and encouraged her to start reading through the literature packet to begin understanding the disease and the implications for David and her family.

It is now two days later and you ask David's mother whether she has had time to read the material you gave her and if she has any questions. She produces the booklets and says she has started reading them. She admits to you that she is a slow reader and has only gotten through the first few pages of the first booklet. When you ask her if she has any questions so far, she opens the booklet and asks what a certain sentence means. You can tell by the way she slowly and phonetically sounds out several words that her reading ability is at a very elementary level. You are suddenly aware that the teaching material you have given her assumes at least a grade 10 reading ability and is much too difficult for her to understand. You realize that during the time until David is discharged you will have to find alternative ways to explain David's illness to her and for teaching her how to take care of her son.

1 Plan your search strategy ahead of time

2 Break down your search topic into components

Because the hospital where you work has no other teaching material for you to use, you decide to search for other resources. You wonder if there are videos or other audiovisual materials that might be utilized. You hope to find articles that describe methods of teaching clients. Decide on the keywords, synonyms, or related terms of your search. The diagram below shows the terms you should have considered. They have been grouped to make the searching process easier.

What are the keywords, synonyms, or related terms?
- cystic fibrosis + education
- health education • teaching methods

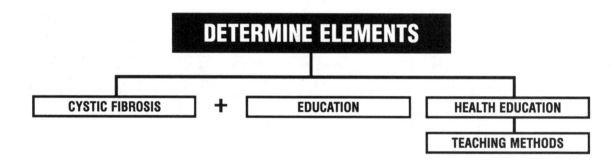

3 Check for subject headings in the Subject Heading List of the CINAHL® database

The following chart displays the subject headings exactly as they appear in the CINAHL Thesaurus.

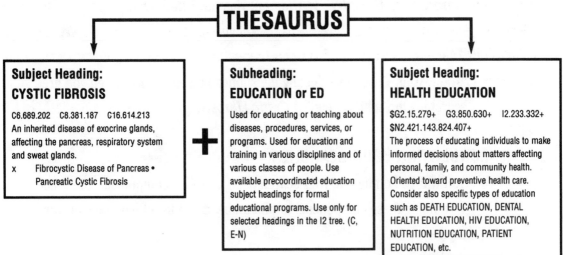

THESAURUS

Subject Heading:
CYSTIC FIBROSIS

C6.689.202   C8.381.187   C16.614.213
An inherited disease of exocrine glands, affecting the pancreas, respiratory system and sweat glands.
x   Fibrocystic Disease of Pancreas •
      Pancreatic Cystic Fibrosis

+

Subheading:
EDUCATION or ED

Used for educating or teaching about diseases, procedures, services, or programs. Used for education and training in various disciplines and of various classes of people. Use available precoordinated education subject headings for formal educational programs. Use only for selected headings in the I2 tree. (C, E-N)

Subject Heading:
HEALTH EDUCATION

$G2.15.279+   G3.850.630+   I2.233.332+
$N2.421.143.824.407+
The process of educating individuals to make informed decisions about matters affecting personal, family, and community health. Oriented toward preventive health care. Consider also specific types of education such as DEATH EDUCATION, DENTAL HEALTH EDUCATION, HIV EDUCATION, NUTRITION EDUCATION, PATIENT EDUCATION, etc.
see also HEALTH EDUCATORS
x   Community Health Education •
      Education, Health

Subject Heading:
TEACHING METHODS

$I2.903.859+
Year: 1983
Ways of presenting materials or conducting instructional activities.

4 Decide which operators and limits you need

A OPERATORS

- Use operator "OR" to connect synonymous or related terms – for example, *Health Education* OR *Teaching Methods*.

- Use operator "AND" to connect the different components – for example, *Cystic Fibrosis* AND (*Health Education* OR *Teaching Methods*).

B LIMITS

- Modify your search by selecting the subheading *education* when you are searching the subject heading *Cystic Fibrosis*.

C CONDUCTING YOUR SEARCHES

- You will be conducting your search using separate components and then combining these components to obtain the actual list of materials on your topic.

  1 The first term you will search is *Cystic Fibrosis*. You will modify the search by selecting the subheading *education*.

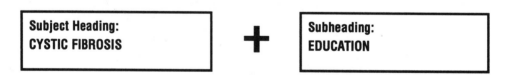

2 The next group of terms you will search is *Health Education – Teaching Methods*.

When you search *Health Education* and *Teaching Methods* select the broad headings and all the specific terms under them by choosing the "explode" option.

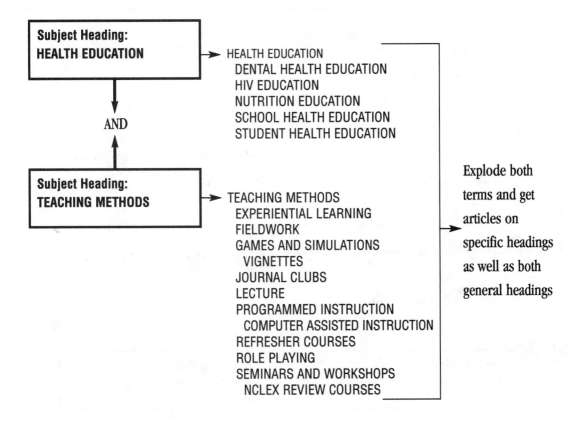

Subject Heading:
HEALTH EDUCATION

AND

Subject Heading:
TEACHING METHODS

HEALTH EDUCATION
   DENTAL HEALTH EDUCATION
   HIV EDUCATION
   NUTRITION EDUCATION
   SCHOOL HEALTH EDUCATION
   STUDENT HEALTH EDUCATION

TEACHING METHODS
   EXPERIENTIAL LEARNING
   FIELDWORK
   GAMES AND SIMULATIONS
    VIGNETTES
   JOURNAL CLUBS
   LECTURE
   PROGRAMMED INSTRUCTION
    COMPUTER ASSISTED INSTRUCTION
   REFRESHER COURSES
   ROLE PLAYING
   SEMINARS AND WORKSHOPS
    NCLEX REVIEW COURSES

Explode both terms and get articles on specific headings as well as both general headings

3 Finally, combine the components using the operator "AND".

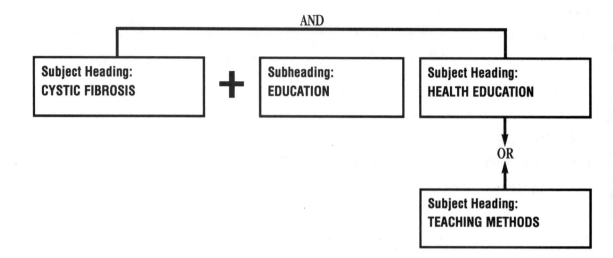

5   Run your search

6   View the results

NOTES

CASE STUDY 9

You are a new graduate from a BSN program and looking for your first job as a registered nurse. You did well in all your coursework, have a solid resume documenting your skills and achievements from your clinicals, and have excellent references. In addition, you worked for 10 years as a special education school teacher before you decided to become a nurse. Unfortunately, due to staffing changes brought about by managed care, RNs are being laid off and more nursing assistants are being hired. The same is true throughout the region where you live, resulting in an overabundance of RNs.

The employment situation for new RNs is bleak. Hospitals everywhere are stating that they are not hiring or that at least one year of experience is required. Still, you have submitted applications to every hospital within driving distance and have requested informational interviews with nurse managers and human resources department personnel. They have all indicated they would love to hire you, but you lack the year of experience they are requiring for employment at this time.

1 Plan your search strategy ahead of time

2 Break down your search topic into components

You know, however, that some new nursing graduates have gotten jobs. When you have asked them how they got those jobs, they have said, "Oh, it was luck." You are frustrated and confused about what more you can do to secure employment as an RN. You decide to search the literature for tips on finding a job in the current job market. You hope to find guidance on to how to make connections with the "right" people. You wonder if your resume and cover letters might be improved. Perhaps there is a way of presenting your years of teaching experience that can make up for your lack of work experience as a nurse. Decide on the keywords, synonyms, or related terms of your search. The diagram below shows the terms you should have considered. They have been grouped together to make the searching process easier.

What are the keywords, synonyms, or related terms?

- new graduate nurses
- job application • employment • job interviews

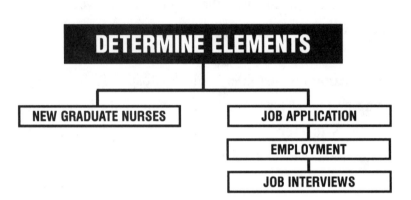

3 Check for subject headings in the Subject Heading List of the CINAHL® database

The following chart displays the subject headings exactly as they appear in the CINAHL Thesaurus.

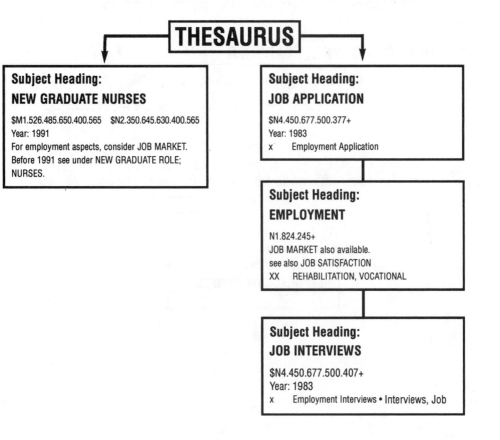

THESAURUS

Subject Heading:
NEW GRADUATE NURSES

$M1.526.485.650.400.565 $N2.350.645.630.400.565
Year: 1991
For employment aspects, consider JOB MARKET.
Before 1991 see under NEW GRADUATE ROLE;
NURSES.

Subject Heading:
JOB APPLICATION

$N4.450.677.500.377+
Year: 1983
x   Employment Application

Subject Heading:
EMPLOYMENT

N1.824.245+
JOB MARKET also available.
see also JOB SATISFACTION
XX   REHABILITATION, VOCATIONAL

Subject Heading:
JOB INTERVIEWS

$N4.450.677.500.407+
Year: 1983
x   Employment Interviews • Interviews, Job

4 Decide which operators you need

A OPERATORS

- Use operator "OR" to connect synonymous or related terms – for example, *Employment* OR *Job Application*.
- Use operator "AND" to connect the different components.

B CONDUCTING YOUR SEARCHES

- You will be conducting your search using separate components and then combining these components to obtain the actual list of materials on your topic.

1 The first heading you will search for is *New Graduate Nurses*.

```
Subject Heading:
NEW GRADUATE NURSES
```

2 The second group of terms you will search for is *Job Application – Employment – Job Interviews*. When you search these three terms select them and all the specific terms under them by choosing the "explode" option.

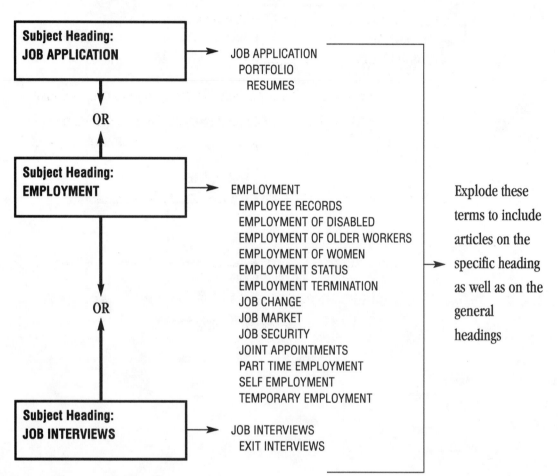

| Subject Heading:
JOB APPLICATION | → | JOB APPLICATION
PORTFOLIO
RESUMES |

OR

| Subject Heading:
EMPLOYMENT | → | EMPLOYMENT
EMPLOYEE RECORDS
EMPLOYMENT OF DISABLED
EMPLOYMENT OF OLDER WORKERS
EMPLOYMENT OF WOMEN
EMPLOYMENT STATUS
EMPLOYMENT TERMINATION
JOB CHANGE
JOB MARKET
JOB SECURITY
JOINT APPOINTMENTS
PART TIME EMPLOYMENT
SELF EMPLOYMENT
TEMPORARY EMPLOYMENT |

OR

| Subject Heading:
JOB INTERVIEWS | → | JOB INTERVIEWS
EXIT INTERVIEWS |

Explode these terms to include articles on the specific heading as well as on the general headings

3 Finally, combine the components using the operator "AND".

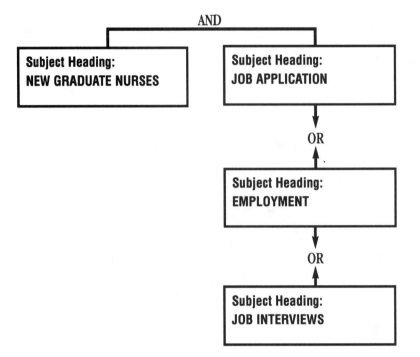

5 Run your search

6 View the results

NOTES

CASE STUDY 10

You are a nurse working on coronary care unit (CCU). The majority of your patients have undergone coronary artery bypass grafts (CABG) or percutaneous transluminal coronary angioplasty (PTCA) procedures. You have noticed that although your hospital is known for serving the Medicaid population, you have very few people with Medicaid on your unit.

You are curious about the economics of who gets these lifesaving, although expensive, procedures. You decide to do some investigation with other nurses working on different medical and surgical floors in your hospital. According to several of them, they, too, have noticed patients receiving more expensive surgeries tend to be privately insured, even though the majority of their patients are on Medicaid.

1 Plan your search strategy ahead of time

2 Break down your search topic into components

This information deeply troubles you. You decide to learn more about the ethical dilemmas posed by the economic realities of modern healthcare delivery. Some of the questions which guide your literature search include: What are the ethical guidelines for rationing treatment? How do the nursing values of equality and justice correspond to the need on the part of providers and administrators to conduct cost/benefit analyses in determining who gets what kind of care? Is it right for a middle-aged, employed, well-insured woman with coronary artery disease to get a bypass while an older, homeless, uninsured man with the same disease gets some medication and told to change his stressful, unhealthy lifestyle? How old, or how poor, must a person be before it no longer makes sense to perform an expensive life-prolonging procedure? How can you as a nurse get involved in the debate on these ethical questions at your hospital? Decide on the keywords, synonyms, or related terms of your search. The diagram below shows the terms you should have considered. They have been grouped together to make the searching process easier.

What are the keywords, synonyms, or related terms?
- ethics, nursing • decision making, ethical
- health resource allocation • economic value of life

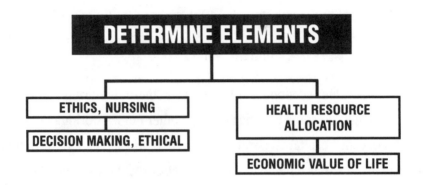

3 Check for subject headings in the Subject Heading List of the CINAHL® database

The following chart displays the subject headings exactly as they appear in the CINAHL Thesaurus.

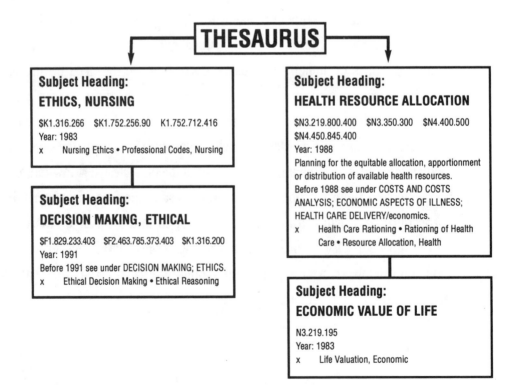

4 Decide which operators you need

A OPERATORS

- Use operator "OR" to connect synonymous or related terms – for example, *Ethics, Nursing* OR *Decision Making, Ethical*.
- Use operator "AND" to connect the different components.

B CONDUCTING YOUR SEARCHES

- You will be conducting your search using separate components and then combining these components to obtain the actual list of materials on your topic.

1 The first group of terms you will search for is *Ethics, Nursing – Decision Making, Ethical*.

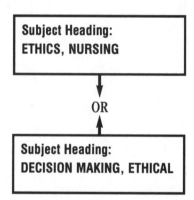

2 The second group of terms you will search for will be *Health Resource Allocation – Economic Value of Life*.

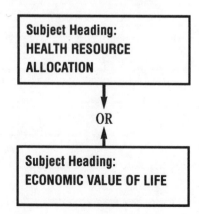

3 Finally, combine the components using the operator "AND".

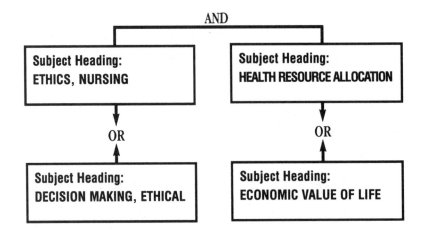

5   Run your search

6   View the results

NOTES

CASE STUDY 11

You are a nurse working in an ambulatory care surgi-center. People come to the center the morning of their surgeries and are discharged to their homes by evening. It is a fast paced environment. Although you sometimes feel frustrated that you don't get to spend enough time with patients and their families, you know people would rather return home quickly to their families than spend time in a hospital.

Most patients come to the surgi-center alone or with one other family member. The majority of these family members leave after the patient is admitted and return when the patient is ready to be discharged. There is, however, a small family waiting room for those who wish to stay.

Recently there have been some problems at the surgi-center. During the last few years your city has seen an increase in the number of immigrants from eastern European countries. Many of these people have Gypsy ancestry. When people from this ethnic group come to the surgi-center, they bring their whole family – parents, spouses, children, grandchildren, sometimes even uncles and aunts. It's not unusual to have 10-15 people from the extended family accompanying a single patient. Furthermore, they all stay at the surgi-center the whole day until the patient is ready to be discharged. During this time these family members fill up the waiting room, spill out onto the street, and sometimes even bring along equipment to cook their meals in the parking lot.

Efforts by the surgi-center administrators to reduce the problem have included posting large signs saying that only two family members per patient are allowed to wait at the center and making sure that pre-op instructions given the day before the surgery include mentioning the limit on the number of family who may accompany the patient. These efforts have not had any result. There is talk among surgi-center staff about the need for security guards to enforce the new "two family members per patient" policy.

1 Plan your search strategy ahead of time

2 Break down your search topic into components

You are concerned that the cultural needs of these patients and their families are not being taken into account. You would like to be able to suggest alternative ways of dealing with the disruptions caused by these families, so you decide to search the literature. First, you need to learn more about their culture. You also need to refresh your memory on conducting cultural assessments of families. Then you hope to find information on bridging differences between traditional health care systems and people of different cultures. You also want to look for anecdotal accounts of how other health institutions have dealt with patients whose values and practices regarding family participation clash with their policies. Decide on the keywords, synonyms, or related terms of your search. The diagram below shows the terms you should have considered. They have been grouped to make the searching easier.

What are the keywords, synonyms, or related terms?

- gypsies
- transcultural care • transcultural nursing

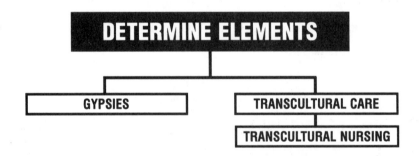

3 Check for subject headings in the Subject Heading List of the CINAHL® database

The following chart displays the subject headings exactly as they appear in the CINAHL Thesaurus.

THESAURUS

Subject Heading:
GYPSIES

$I1.76.250.416.280   I1.880.143.522.282   M1.194.265
Year: 1997
Before 1997 see under TRANSIENTS AND MIGRANTS.

Subject Heading:
TRANSCULTURAL CARE

$E2.760.940
Year: 1993
see also CULTURE BROKERAGE (IOWA NIC)

Subject Heading:
TRANSCULTURAL NURSING

$N2.421.533.910
A nurse within own country, providing care to patients of other cultures. For discussions of the nurse practicing in the health care system of another country, see INTERNATIONAL NURSING. see also HEALTH SERVICES, INDIGENOUS • TRANSCULTURAL NURSING SOCIETY

4 Decide which operators you need

A OPERATORS

- Use operator "OR" to connect synonymous or related terms – for example, *Transcultural Care* OR *Transcultural Nursing*.
- Use operator "AND" to connect the different components.

B CONDUCTING YOUR SEARCHES

- You will be conducting your search using separate components and then combining these components to obtain the actual list of materials on your topic.

    1   The first term you will search for is *Gypsies*. Since this term was added in 1997 the results will not retrieve material indexed before 1997 (see history note).

Subject Heading:
GYPSIES

2 The second group of terms you will search for is *Transcultural Care – Transcultural Nursing*.

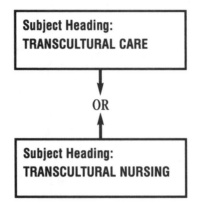

3 Finally, combine the components using the operator "AND".

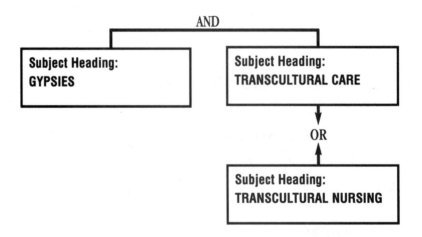

5   Run your search

6   View the results

NOTES

CASE STUDY 12

You are the director of an outpatient cardiac rehabilitation program. Your clients are primarily coronary artery disease (CAD) patients. They may have had an acute myocardial infarction, or may have undergone a procedure such as coronary artery bypass graft (CABG) or percutaneous transluminal coronary angioplasty (PTCA). Some of them have diffuse, inoperable disease. Your program has a multi-pronged approach to lifestyle modification and CAD risk reduction. It consists of a structured exercise program, a stop-smoking program, consultations in nutrition and diet, and yoga/meditation groups for stress reduction. There are weekly educational lectures and weekly support groups for dealing with the complex psychological issues surrounding the diagnosis of heart disease.

The administrators at your hospital are evaluating whether your program is cost-effective. You have shown them the research which indicates that cardiac rehabilitation reduces the incidence of future MIs in people who have already had an MI, and reduces the rate of re-stenosis in people who have had a CABG or PTCA. You have documented that your program is similar to those of the studies which demonstrated this cost-effectiveness. Yet, your program is being threatened because of the hospital's need to cut costs. Certain administrators do not believe your program significantly reduces the long-term rehospitalization rates of the specific cardiac patients seen at your hospital.

You realize that in order to continue your program, you need to produce data specifically on your hospital's cardiac patients. You know from your experience in working with your clients that being in the cardiac rehab program improves their quality of life, but you need to prove whether or not it is cost-effective for the hospital in the long term. Before you begin gathering your data, however, you need to know exactly what information you should collect and in what format the data should be collected. You know that you need to collect information such as patient age, sex, diagnosis, complications and length of time in the cardiac rehab program, but you want to make sure you don't miss other important categories. You have some knowledge of computer databases and remember basic statistical methods from nursing school, but you want to find the best way to store data so it can be easily retrieved for analysis.

1 Plan your search strategy ahead of time

2 Break down your search topic into components

You decide to search the literature for guidance in managing the information you will be collecting. Decide on the keywords, synonyms, or related terms of your search. The diagram below shows the terms you should have considered. They have been grouped to make the searching easier.

What are the keywords, synonyms, or related terms?

- database construction • database management software • data management •
- data analysis software • data analysis, computer assisted

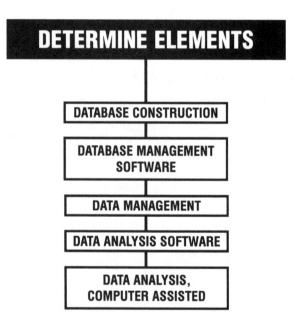

3 Check for subject headings in the Subject Heading List of the CINAHL® database

The following chart displays the subject headings exactly as they appear in the CINAHL Thesaurus.

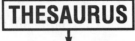

THESAURUS

Subject Heading:

DATABASE CONSTRUCTION

$L1.328.220.395.370
Year: 1991
see also DATABASES
XX   DATA WAREHOUSE

Subject Heading:

DATABASE MANAGEMENT SOFTWARE

$L1.328.220.312.810.350
Year: 1986
Before 1986 see under COMPUTER PROGRAMS.
XX   DATA MANAGEMENT

Subject Heading:

DATA MANAGEMENT

$L1.328.290+
Year: 1997
The process of analyzing and defining what data is
to be collected, determining the procedures needed
to effectively collect data, and the actual collection of
data to produce the required information.
see also DATABASE MANAGEMENT SOFTWARE.

Subject Heading:

DATA ANALYSIS SOFTWARE

$L1.328.220.312.810.300
Year: 1993
Before 1993 see under DATA ANALYSIS; SOFTWARE.
x   Statistical Software
XX   DATA ANALYSIS, COMPUTER ASSISTED

Subject Heading:

DATA ANALYSIS, COMPUTER ASSISTED

$H1.770.644.600.280.280 $L1.328.220.395.320
Year: 1997
The use of computers to collect and assist in the
analysis of data. Consider also SIGNAL
PROCESSING, COMPUTER ASSISTED.
see also DATA ANALYSIS SOFTWARE
x   Computer Assisted Data Analysis

---

4 Decide which operators and limits you need

A OPERATORS

- Use operator "OR" to connect synonymous or related terms – for example, *Database Construction* OR *Database Management Software* OR *Data Management* OR *Data Analysis Software* OR *Data Analysis, Computer Assisted*.

B LIMITS

- Since each specific term will retrieve a large number of articles you need to restrict your search terms to focus. Also limit your search to the last five years.

C CONDUCTING YOUR SEARCHES

- You will be conducting your search using separate components and then connecting these components to obtain the actual list of materials on your topic.

  1 The terms that you will search for are *Database Construction – Database Management Software – Data Management – Data Analysis Software – Data Analysis, Computer Assisted*.

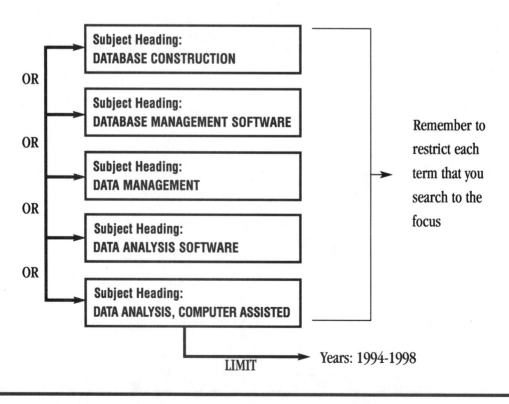

5 Run your search

6 View the results

NOTES

CASE STUDY 13

You are the director of a hospice program which serves people with AIDS. The agency has been in existence since the beginning of the AIDS epidemic and has a solid reputation among AIDS organizations and service providers as a place where patients and families receive the highest quality care. The program includes both a residential component for those who cannot stay in their own homes or who are homeless, as well as visiting nurses who care for patients in their own homes.

Because grant money for AIDS programs has been slowly diminishing, it has become more difficult to find the funds to operate your agency. You have begun looking at ways in which your agency can serve other populations, and thus be eligible for other sources of funding. You have learned that there is a need in your city for a pediatric hospice program. You and members of your board of directors have met with people from community agencies that serve the needs of families with children who have cancer, and with administrators from the University Hospital in your city which is nationally known in pediatric oncology. Representatives from these organizations have expressed interest in establishing a collaborative relationship with your agency to develop a pediatric hospice program.

You are now getting ready to have a meeting with your staff in which you want to present the idea of expanding your hospice services to include the pediatric population. You anticipate that this may generate strong negative reactions among your hospice nurses. You decide to do some research to prepare yourself for answering their objections. You suspect they will raise the fact that pediatric hospices usually allow aggressive medical treatments to continue until the patient dies, whereas your agency's current philosophy is that only palliative treatment is given. You also suspect they will claim that they are not trained to deal with the different family dynamics when the dying patient is still a child.

1 Plan your search strategy ahead of time

2 Break down your search topic into components

In your literature search you hope to find articles that outline the range of views regarding the scope of hospice philosophies and services, as well as issues that are unique for nurses working with terminally ill children. You hope to find references to other hospice programs so that you can make personal contact with them. In addition, you need to find articles on managing and implementing change in agencies. You want to refresh your memory on different change theories and get ideas for how to present the idea of expanding your agency's services in a way that is most likely to be received positively. Decide on the keywords, synonyms, or related terms of your search. The diagram below shows the terms you should have considered. They have been grouped to make the searching easier.

What are the keywords, synonyms, or related terms?
- hospices • hospice care • hospice nursing
- change theory
- change management • organizational change

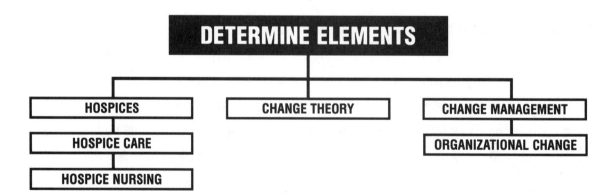

3 Check for subject headings in the Subject Heading List of the CINAHL® database

The following chart displays the subject headings exactly as they appear in the CINAHL Thesaurus.

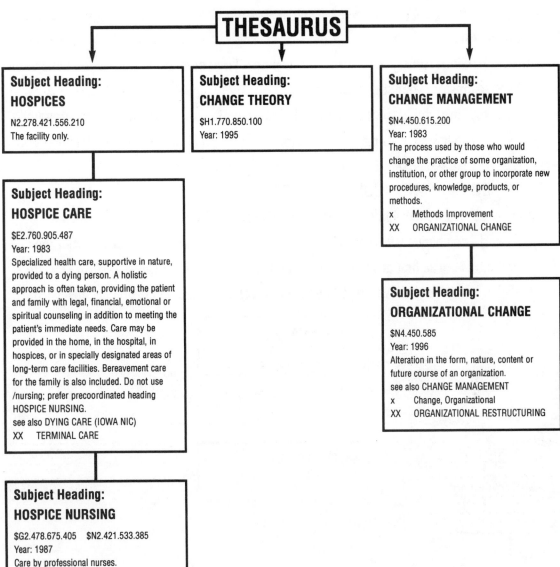

THESAURUS

Subject Heading:
HOSPICES

N2.278.421.556.210
The facility only.

Subject Heading:
CHANGE THEORY

$H1.770.850.100
Year: 1995

Subject Heading:
CHANGE MANAGEMENT

$N4.450.615.200
Year: 1983
The process used by those who would change the practice of some organization, institution, or other group to incorporate new procedures, knowledge, products, or methods.
x   Methods Improvement
XX   ORGANIZATIONAL CHANGE

Subject Heading:
HOSPICE CARE

$E2.760.905.487
Year: 1983
Specialized health care, supportive in nature, provided to a dying person. A holistic approach is often taken, providing the patient and family with legal, financial, emotional or spiritual counseling in addition to meeting the patient's immediate needs. Care may be provided in the home, in the hospital, in hospices, or in specially designated areas of long-term care facilities. Bereavement care for the family is also included. Do not use /nursing; prefer precoordinated heading HOSPICE NURSING.
see also DYING CARE (IOWA NIC)
XX   TERMINAL CARE

Subject Heading:
ORGANIZATIONAL CHANGE

$N4.450.585
Year: 1996
Alteration in the form, nature, content or future course of an organization.
see also CHANGE MANAGEMENT
x   Change, Organizational
XX   ORGANIZATIONAL RESTRUCTURING

Subject Heading:
HOSPICE NURSING

$G2.478.675.405 $N2.421.533.385
Year: 1987
Care by professional nurses.
Before 1987 see under HOSPICE CARE.

4 Decide which operators and limits you need

A OPERATORS

- Use operator "OR" to connect synonymous or related terms – for example, *Hospices* OR *Hospice Care* OR *Hospice Nursing*.

- Use operator "AND" to connect the different components – for example, *Change Management* AND *Organizational Change*.

B LIMITS

- Since each specific term will retrieve a large number of articles you need to restrict your search to focus.

- Since the hospice program will be expanding to the pediatric population limit your search using the population groups *infant, child-preschool, child*, and *adolescence*.

C CONDUCTING YOUR SEARCHES

- You will be conducting your search using separate components and then combining these components to obtain the actual list of materials on your topic.

  1 The first group of terms you will search for is *Hospices – Hospice Care – Hospice Nursing*. Limit your search using the population groups listed above.

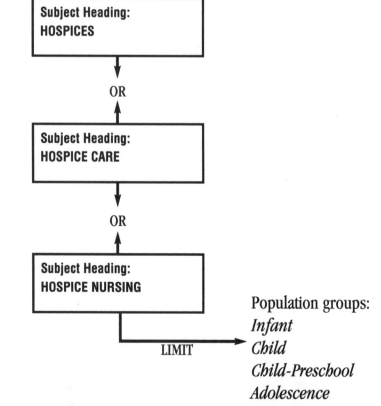

2 The second search will be for the term *Change Theory*.

Subject Heading:
CHANGE THEORY

3 The third group of terms you will search for is *Change Management –
Organizational Change*.

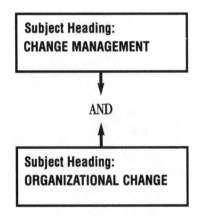

4 Finally, combine the components using both the "AND" and "OR" operators.

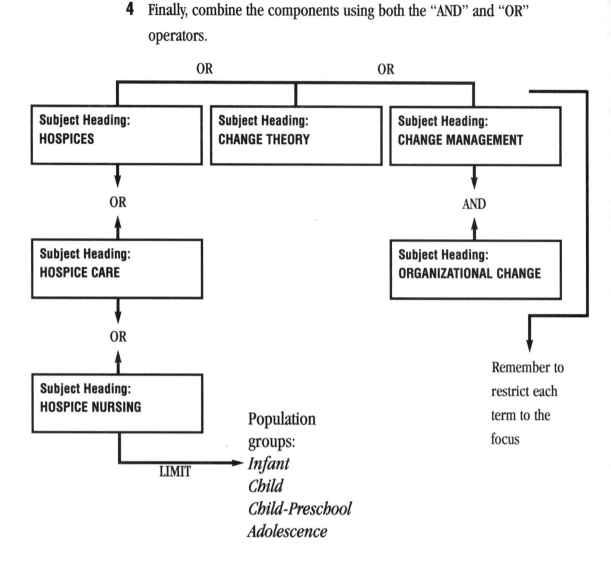

5   Run your search

6   View the results

NOTES

CASE STUDY 14

You are a nurse working at an outpatient psychiatric clinic. Geraldine, a 58 year old client with bipolar disorder, has been served by the clinic since it began 20 years ago. When she adheres to her medication regimen (lithium, 300 mg PO QID), she is able to take care of herself and actively participate in the lives of her husband, children, and grandchildren. As with many people with bipolar disorder, Geraldine has a history of discontinuing her medication when she feels like she is functioning normally. Her general pattern has been that after stopping her medication she has a manic episode lasting 1-2 weeks. This is followed by a plunge into suicidal depression which necessitates her admission to the inpatient psychiatric unit. It usually takes 3 weeks to stabilize her again so that she can be discharged to her home. This pattern is repeated several times a year.

You know from your previous work with Geraldine's husband, Bill, that he is not helpful in ensuring her medication compliance. He reports that at the beginning of her manic phases she becomes "the woman I married. She laughs and sings and is full of energy again. She busies herself in the garden and bakes endless amount of cookies and cakes which she gives to all the neighbors. And we even make love again." Bill identifies himself as a deeply religious man who believes if he just has enough faith, God will cure his wife. He admits that each time she stops taking her medication, he hopes this time Geraldine will be cured. Each time, however, the cycle repeats itself – Geraldine eventually spins manically out of control, goes into a deep depression, and eventually needs to be rehospitalized.

Geraldine is supposed to come to your clinic every month to have her serum lithium level tested. She did not show up for her scheduled appointment today, even though you confirmed it with her just last week. You suspect she has stopped taking her lithium again and may be entering her manic phase. In the past when this has happened, you have tried to contact Bill to encourage him to bring her into the clinic. This has usually led to his claim that she has been cured and doesn't need the medication or your services any more. Before you contact him this time, you want to develop a new intervention/teaching plan.

1 Plan your search strategy ahead of time

2 Break down your search topic into components

You decide to search the literature for methods to help both Geraldine and Bill comply with her medication regimen. Your goal is to break the cycle so that Geraldine won't need to be hospitalized several times a year. Decide on the keywords, synonyms, or related terms of your search. The diagram below shows the terms you should have considered. They have been grouped to make the searching process easier.

What are the keywords, synonyms, or related terms?
- patient education • teaching methods
- patient compliance • self administration

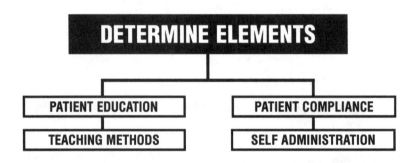

3 Check for subject headings in the Subject Heading List of the CINAHL® database

The following chart displays the subject headings exactly as they appear in the CINAHL Thesaurus.

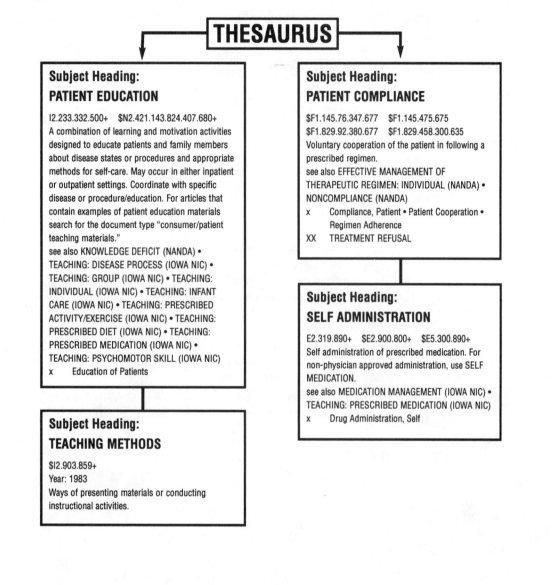

THESAURUS

Subject Heading:
PATIENT EDUCATION

I2.233.332.500+ $N2.421.143.824.407.680+
A combination of learning and motivation activities designed to educate patients and family members about disease states or procedures and appropriate methods for self-care. May occur in either inpatient or outpatient settings. Coordinate with specific disease or procedure/education. For articles that contain examples of patient education materials search for the document type "consumer/patient teaching materials."
see also KNOWLEDGE DEFICIT (NANDA) • TEACHING: DISEASE PROCESS (IOWA NIC) • TEACHING: GROUP (IOWA NIC) • TEACHING: INDIVIDUAL (IOWA NIC) • TEACHING: INFANT CARE (IOWA NIC) • TEACHING: PRESCRIBED ACTIVITY/EXERCISE (IOWA NIC) • TEACHING: PRESCRIBED DIET (IOWA NIC) • TEACHING: PRESCRIBED MEDICATION (IOWA NIC) • TEACHING: PSYCHOMOTOR SKILL (IOWA NIC)
x   Education of Patients

Subject Heading:
TEACHING METHODS

$I2.903.859+
Year: 1983
Ways of presenting materials or conducting instructional activities.

Subject Heading:
PATIENT COMPLIANCE

$F1.145.76.347.677 $F1.145.475.675
$F1.829.92.380.677 $F1.829.458.300.635
Voluntary cooperation of the patient in following a prescribed regimen.
see also EFFECTIVE MANAGEMENT OF THERAPEUTIC REGIMEN: INDIVIDUAL (NANDA) • NONCOMPLIANCE (NANDA)
x   Compliance, Patient • Patient Cooperation • Regimen Adherence
XX   TREATMENT REFUSAL

Subject Heading:
SELF ADMINISTRATION

E2.319.890+ $E2.900.800+ $E5.300.890+
Self administration of prescribed medication. For non-physician approved administration, use SELF MEDICATION.
see also MEDICATION MANAGEMENT (IOWA NIC) • TEACHING: PRESCRIBED MEDICATION (IOWA NIC)
x   Drug Administration, Self

4 Decide which operators you need

A OPERATORS

- Use operator "OR" to connect synonymous or related terms – for example, *Patient Education* OR *Teaching Methods*.

- Use operator "AND" to connect the different components.

B CONDUCTING YOUR SEARCHES

- You will be conducting your search using separate components and then combining these components to obtain the actual list of materials on your topic.

1 The first group of terms you will search for is *Patient Education – Teaching Methods*.

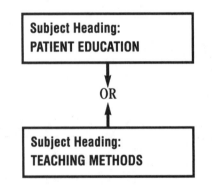

2 The second group of terms you will search for is *Patient Compliance – Self Administration*.

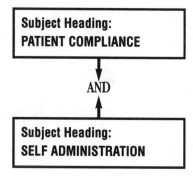

3 Finally, combine the components using the operator "AND".

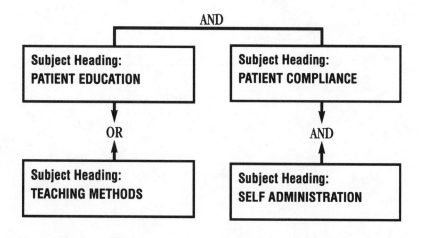

5   Run your search

6   View the results

NOTES

CASE STUDY 15

You are a nursing student beginning your maternity rotation. You have seen several videos on childbirth, including one that showed women from South America delivering in a squatting position. During your initial orientation to the birthing rooms on your unit, the head nurse explains that the birthing bed can be taken apart to allow the patient to squat. She adds, however, that "no one ever wants to do that, and we don't encourage it because it means rearranging the furniture."

You know from your study of the demographics in your city that there is a large immigrant population from several South American countries. In fact, the first delivery in which you assist is with Maria, a young woman who just arrived in the U.S. from Bolivia. You notice that several times during her second stage of labor she attempts to get up. Maria knows almost no English, and no one in the room speaks more than a few words of Spanish. Each time she attempts to get off the bed the nurse you are working with tells her to lie down again and rest between contractions. You wonder whether she is attempting to assume a squatting position for the final delivery.

1 Plan your search strategy ahead of time

2 Break down your search topic into components

You want to learn more about different positions and methods of childbirth. You also want to know if anything has been written on the psychological impact on laboring women when health professionals prevent them from following their traditional customs. You are curious about how medical institutions which serve many diverse cultures can adapt their services and facilities to better meet patient needs. Decide on the keywords, synonyms, or related terms of your search. The diagram below shows the terms you should have considered. They have been grouped to make the searching process easier.

What are the keywords, synonyms, or related terms?

- birthing positions • childbirth + methods
- transcultural care • transcultural nursing • cultural sensitivity
- childbirth

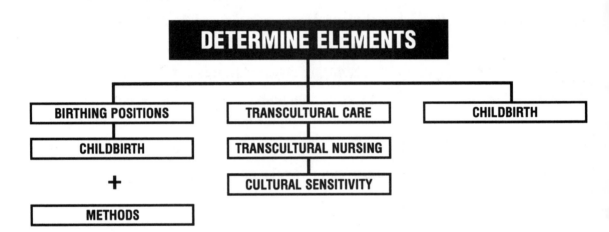

3 Check for subject headings in the Subject Heading List of the CINAHL® database

The following chart displays the subject headings exactly as they appear in the CINAHL Thesaurus.

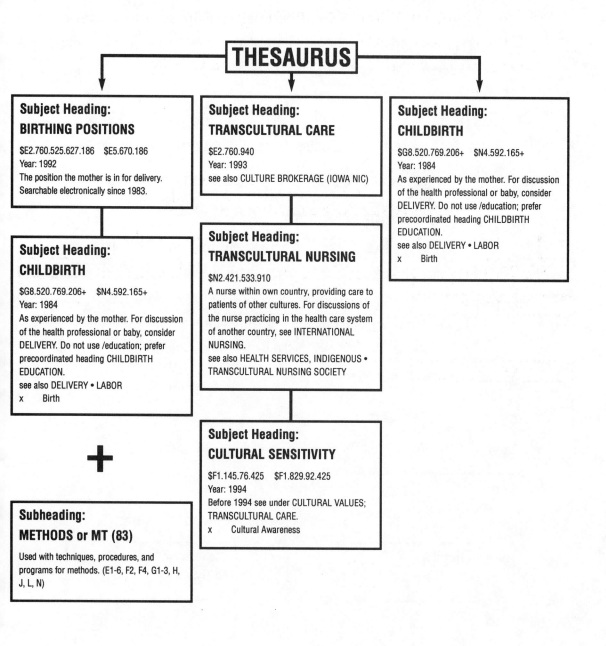

THESAURUS

Subject Heading:
BIRTHING POSITIONS

$E2.760.525.627.186 $E5.670.186
Year: 1992
The position the mother is in for delivery.
Searchable electronically since 1983.

Subject Heading:
TRANSCULTURAL CARE

$E2.760.940
Year: 1993
see also CULTURE BROKERAGE (IOWA NIC)

Subject Heading:
CHILDBIRTH

$G8.520.769.206+ $N4.592.165+
Year: 1984
As experienced by the mother. For discussion of the health professional or baby, consider DELIVERY. Do not use /education; prefer precoordinated heading CHILDBIRTH EDUCATION.
see also DELIVERY • LABOR
x   Birth

Subject Heading:
CHILDBIRTH

$G8.520.769.206+ $N4.592.165+
Year: 1984
As experienced by the mother. For discussion of the health professional or baby, consider DELIVERY. Do not use /education; prefer precoordinated heading CHILDBIRTH EDUCATION.
see also DELIVERY • LABOR
x   Birth

Subject Heading:
TRANSCULTURAL NURSING

$N2.421.533.910
A nurse within own country, providing care to patients of other cultures. For discussions of the nurse practicing in the health care system of another country, see INTERNATIONAL NURSING.
see also HEALTH SERVICES, INDIGENOUS • TRANSCULTURAL NURSING SOCIETY

+

Subject Heading:
CULTURAL SENSITIVITY

$F1.145.76.425 $F1.829.92.425
Year: 1994
Before 1994 see under CULTURAL VALUES; TRANSCULTURAL CARE.
x   Cultural Awareness

Subheading:
METHODS or MT (83)

Used with techniques, procedures, and programs for methods. (E1-6, F2, F4, G1-3, H, J, L, N)

4 Decide which operators and limits you need

A OPERATORS

- Use operator "OR" to connect synonymous or related terms – for example, *Birthing Positions* OR *Childbirth*.

- Use operator "AND" to connect the different components – for example (*Transcultural Care* OR *Transcultural Nursing* OR *Cultural Sensitivity*) AND (*Childbirth*).

B LIMITS

- Modify your search by selecting the subheading *methods* when you are searching the subject heading *Childbirth*.

C CONDUCTING YOUR SEARCHES

- You will be conducting your search using separate components and then combining these components to obtain the actual list of materials on your topic.

1 The first group of terms you will search for is *Birthing Positions – Childbirth*. You will modify the search on *Childbirth* by selecting the subheading *methods*.

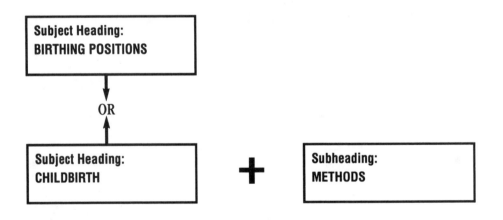

2 The second group of terms you will search for is *Transcultural Care –
Transcultural Nursing – Cultural Sensitivity*.

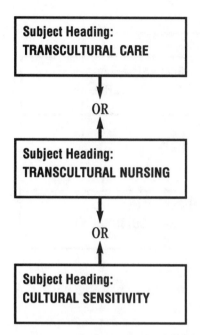

3 Then search for *Childbirth*.

> **Subject Heading:**
> **CHILDBIRTH**

4 Finally, combine the components using both the "AND" and "OR" operators.

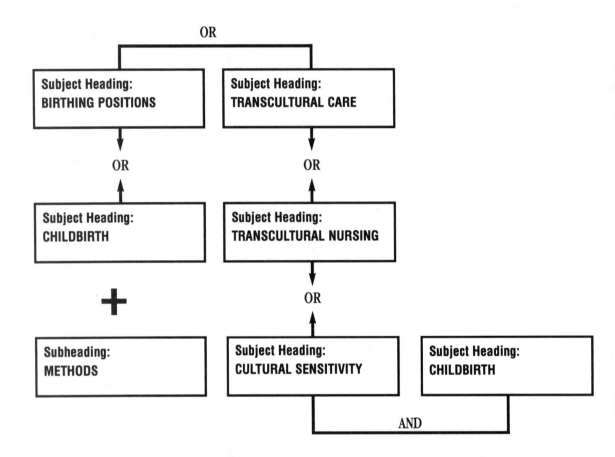

5   Run your search

6   View the results

NOTES

CASE STUDY 16

Mrs. Simon is one of your patients in the nursing home where you just started working. From reading her chart and talking with other nurses, you learn that she has lived at your facility for almost 10 years and is now 89 years old. She was first admitted when she had a cerebral vascular accident (CVA) that left her unable to care for herself or her husband, who was blind. Since her admission, her family and social resources slowly slipped away. First her husband died, then both of her children moved away because of job relocation. She used to have grandchildren who visited occasionally, but they haven't been by to see her in over four years. All of her friends in the community have died or gone to live in other nursing homes, and the few friends she made at the nursing home when she was first admitted have also died.

Mrs. Simon's physical condition has also deteriorated dramatically over the years. A second stroke 5 years ago left her confined to a wheelchair and incontinent of both urine and stool. She has had several hospital admissions for pneumonia, each bout leaving her weaker and more frail. For the past six months her legs have become too contracted to set her up in a chair, and she has developed stage III pressure ulcers on her sacrum and right heel. Because of progressive weight loss, two weeks ago the doctor ordered the insertion of a nasogastric tube with instructions to tube feed her Ensure® if she eats less than 50% of her meal.

You first meet Mrs. Simon when you make the initial check on all your patients. You greet her with a smile and ask how she slept that night. She stares blankly back at you and says, "I just want to die." You offer her a consoling touch and let her know that you will be one of her regular nurses who will be around if she would like to talk more about her feelings. During the next few days you carry out your routine care with Mrs. Simon – bathing, dressing changes on her pressure ulcers, medications, tube feedings. With each encounter Mrs. Simon pleads, "Don't do that, just let me die." When you ask her why she wants to die, she responds by describing all the losses in her life. She tells of having lived an active and fulfilling life and states that the condition she is in now is worse than death. She says the doctors and nurses all say she is simply depressed and should be grateful for the good care she is getting. She grabs your hand and again pleads with you to just let her die.

You feel overwhelmed. Although you agree with other nursing home personnel that Mrs. Simon has a depressed mood, you also sense that she has a rational, heart-felt desire to end her life. Although you are committed to helping people live as long and as comfortably as possible, you wonder whether the staff should honor Mrs. Simon's request and discontinue all life-sustaining care. Before you approach your supervisor with a recommendation to re-evaluate Mrs. Simon's care plan so that she can be allowed to die, you want to gain more information.

1 Plan your search strategy ahead of time

2 Break down your search topic into components

You decide to do a literature search to find what has been written on the topic of letting elderly people decide to terminate their own care. You want to define your own ethical beliefs in this area, as well as gain insight into the legal nature of the arguments. You hope to find stories from other nurses who have had to make decisions to honor their patients' requests to die. You also want to learn more about how nurses working with the frail elderly can empower them to make such life and death decisions. Decide on the keywords, synonyms, or related terms of your search. The diagram below shows terms you should have considered. They have been grouped to make the searching process easier.

What are the keywords, synonyms, or related terms?

- treatment refusal • right to die

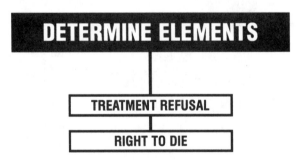

3 Check for subject headings in the Subject Heading List of the CINAHL® database

The following chart displays the subject headings exactly as they appear in the CINAHL Thesaurus.

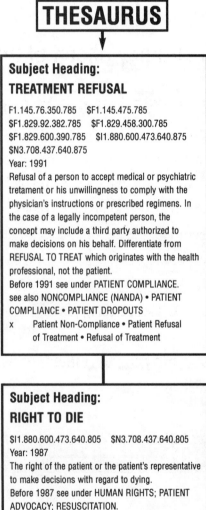

THESAURUS

Subject Heading:
TREATMENT REFUSAL

F1.145.76.350.785 $F1.145.475.785
$F1.829.92.382.785 $F1.829.458.300.785
$F1.829.600.390.785 $I1.880.600.473.640.875
$N3.708.437.640.875
Year: 1991
Refusal of a person to accept medical or psychiatric tretament or his unwillingness to comply with the physician's instructions or prescribed regimens. In the case of a legally incompetent person, the concept may include a third party authorized to make decisions on his behalf. Differentiate from REFUSAL TO TREAT which originates with the health professional, not the patient.
Before 1991 see under PATIENT COMPLIANCE.
see also NONCOMPLIANCE (NANDA) • PATIENT COMPLIANCE • PATIENT DROPOUTS
x   Patient Non-Compliance • Patient Refusal of Treatment • Refusal of Treatment

Subject Heading:
RIGHT TO DIE

$I1.880.600.473.640.805 $N3.708.437.640.805
Year: 1987
The right of the patient or the patient's representative to make decisions with regard to dying.
Before 1987 see under HUMAN RIGHTS; PATIENT ADVOCACY; RESUSCITATION.
x   Death with Dignity
XX   ADVANCE DIRECTIVES

4 Decide which operators and limits you need

A OPERATORS

- Use operator "OR" to connect synonymous or related terms – for example, *Treatment Refusal* OR *Right to Die*.

B LIMITS

- Limit your search by using the population group *aged*.

C CONDUCTING YOUR SEARCHES

- You will be conducting your search using separate components and then combining these components to obtain the actual list of materials on your topic.
- You will search for the terms *Treatment Refusal – Right to Die* and limit by using *aged*.

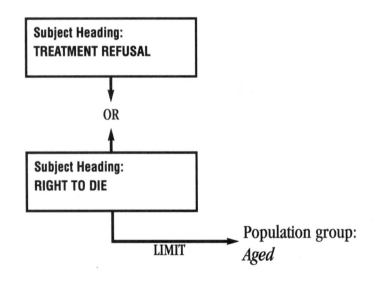

5   Run your search

6   View the results

NOTES

CASE STUDY 17

Sandra is a 28-year-old woman who is a client of your prenatal clinic. She is currently in her fifth month of pregnancy. Following her first visit two months ago when she came in and had a positive pregnancy test, you made the following note in her chart:

"Client is a 28-year-old G1P0 who presents in her 13th week of pregnancy (Nagel's rule). Although pregnancy was not planned, she states 'I really want this baby.' She lives with father of baby and works as retail clerk. Vital signs: T-36.9 °, P-72, R-18, BP-126/68. Current weight: 138 lbs. (5 lbs. above stated pre-pregnant weight). Client has hematoma below R eye which she says resulted from running into cabinet door in kitchen last week. Urinalysis - negative for glucose, 1+ protein. All tests for STDs - negative. Client admits to occasional alcohol use, but states she will stop drinking now that she knows she is pregnant. She has 1 pack/day cig. smoking history since age 16. Client states desire to quit. Other drug history denied. Client given referral for help with smoking cessation. Initial nutritional assessment done and client instructed to take 30 mg iron supplement QD and to increase daily milk intake to 1 L/day."

Since that first visit you have seen Sandra two more times at one-month intervals. Significant data from those visits include BP readings of 138/74 and 152/80 and weights of 143 lbs. and 148 lbs., with 2+ edema in her feet. From these changes, you suspect she may be developing pregnancy-induced hypertension (PIH). You have set up weekly appointments to more closely monitor Sandra's pregnancy. In addition, you have noticed that at each visit Sandra has had new and old bruises on her face and arms. When asked about them, she has dismissed them as resulting from her clumsiness in the kitchen. You suspect, however, that she may be the victim of domestic violence.

Before your visit with Sandra next week, you want to learn more about assessing for physical/emotional/sexual abuse. You know that this is a difficult and sensitive subject to discuss with clients. You have already heard your client's explanation that her bruises are a result of household accidents. Although you have not worked with battered women in the past, you recognize your client exhibits some of the classic signs of being battered. You even realize that the rise in blood pressure and weight gain, which at this point are not high enough for a diagnosis of PIH, could actually be the result of the stress of being battered.

1 Plan your search strategy ahead of time

2 Break down your search topic into components

At this point you do not yet feel you have built a very strong trusting relationship with your client, and you don't want to do anything which might turn her away from your clinic, especially considering that she may be developing PIH. Therefore, you decide to go to the nursing literature to find information on how to approach your client on the topic of being abused. Decide on the keywords, synonyms, or related terms of your search. The diagram below shows the terms you should have considered. They have been grouped together to make the searching process easier.

What are the keywords, synonyms, or related terms?
- partner abuse
- nursing assessment • nursing interventions

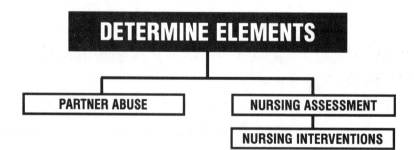

3 Check for subject headings in the Subject Heading List of the CINAHL® database

The following chart displays the subject headings exactly as they appear in the CINAHL Thesaurus.

THESAURUS

Subject Heading:
PARTNER ABUSE

$F3.126.842.89.734.350.690+
$I1.198.240.856.350.690+
$I1.880.735.191.900.350.690+ $I1.880.735.620
Year: 1994
Abuse of one's significant other. Use SPOUSE ABUSE for abuse of one's husband or wife.
Before 1994 see under SPOUSE ABUSE; VIOLENCE.
see also ABUSE PROTECTION (IOWA NIC)

Subject Heading:
NURSING ASSESSMENT

$E1.693 $E1.700.675 $N4.592.450.550.300
Year: 1988
An identification by a nurse of the needs, preferences, and abilities of a patient. Assessment follows an interview with and observation of a patient by the nurse and considers the signs and symptoms of the condition, the patient's verbal and nonverbal communication, medical and social history, and any other information available. It is the first stage of the nursing process.
see also SURVEILLANCE (IOWA NIC)
x   Assessment, Nursing

Subject Heading:
NURSING INTERVENTIONS

$N4.592.450.550.525
Year: 1991
Action based on scientific rationale that is executed to benefit the client in a predicted way related to the nursing diagnosis and the stated goals.
Before 1991 see under NURSING CARE; NURSING PRACTICE.
x   Interventions, Nursing

4 Decide which operators and limits you need

A OPERATORS

- Use operator "OR" to connect synonymous or related terms – for example, *Partner Abuse* AND (*Nursing Assessment* OR *Nursing Interventions*).
- Use operator "AND" to connect the different components.

B LIMITS

- Limit your search using the population group *pregnancy*.

C CONDUCTING YOUR SEARCHES

- Search using the heading *Partner Abuse*. When you search for *Partner Abuse* select it and the specific terms under it by choosing the "explode" option.

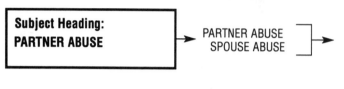

```
┌─────────────────────┐
│ Subject Heading:    │        PARTNER ABUSE          Explode Partner Abuse
│ PARTNER ABUSE       │───▶    SPOUSE ABUSE    ──▶     and get articles on the
│                     │                               specific headings as well
└─────────────────────┘                               as the general heading
                                                       Partner Abuse
```

- Then search for *Nursing Assessment – Nursing Interventions*.

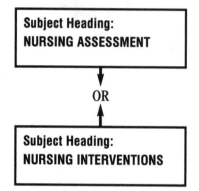

```
┌──────────────────────────┐
│ Subject Heading:         │
│ NURSING ASSESSMENT       │
└──────────────────────────┘
              │
             OR
              ▲
┌──────────────────────────┐
│ Subject Heading:         │
│ NURSING INTERVENTIONS    │
└──────────────────────────┘
```

- Finally, combine the components using the "AND" operator, then limit your search to the population group *pregnancy*.

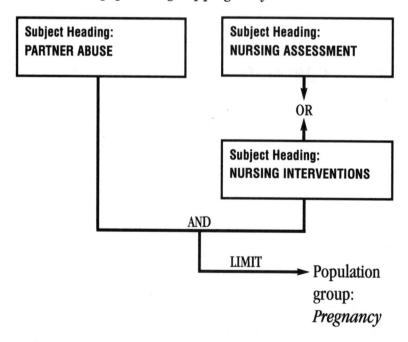

```
┌──────────────────────┐      ┌──────────────────────────┐
│ Subject Heading:     │      │ Subject Heading:         │
│ PARTNER ABUSE        │      │ NURSING ASSESSMENT       │
└──────────────────────┘      └──────────────────────────┘
                                          │
                                         OR
                                          ▲
                              ┌──────────────────────────┐
                              │ Subject Heading:         │
                              │ NURSING INTERVENTIONS    │
                              └──────────────────────────┘

                      AND

                      LIMIT ──────▶  Population
                                     group:
                                     Pregnancy
```

5   Run your search

6   View the results

NOTES

CASE STUDY 18

Tom is a 49-year-old diabetic male who has just been referred to the dialysis unit where you are a case manager. Reviewing Tom's chart you learn that he was diagnosed with insulin-dependent diabetes mellitus (IDDM) at age 5, but that his diabetes has never been well controlled. Although he has been referred to the diabetes clinic numerous times for instruction in managing his disease, he has never made use of their teaching services. Tom has also had hypertension since he was 28. Without medication his blood pressure runs about 160/100 and he admits to not taking his medication because he does not like the side effects. Tom's kidneys began to fail six months ago, and he has deteriorated rapidly since then. He is now in end-stage renal failure, requiring dialysis three times a week.

During your first home visit you discuss with Tom his feelings about needing dialysis and assess whether he understands the severity of his physical condition. "We all die sometime," he states fatalistically. You learn that Tom drinks 6-8 cans of beer a day, smokes 2 packs of cigarettes a day and has a high-salt diet, including a lot of junk food. You ascertain that Tom's main activity is going to the park each day to hang out with a couple of friends. His main priority seems to be securing beer, cigarettes and potato chips for his daily trip to the park. He is angry that on the days he is dialyzed, his whole day is used up and his routine is disrupted.

Tom is on disability and lives with his sister, Maggie, and her family. During your interview with her you learn that Maggie does most of the meal preparation for Tom. She states her frustration in trying to make meals that are healthy, only to see Tom "dump a ton of salt all over his plate." For years she has encouraged him to monitor his blood sugar and take his high blood pressure medicine, but he has always said, "Don't worry about me, I feel fine." Maggie clearly understands that Tom's physical condition is very serious, and feels guilty that she has not done enough to prevent his current situation. "Maybe I could have removed all the salt from the house and made him stop drinking. It's just that since he was injured in that factory accident 10 years ago, I kind of decided he deserved to enjoy life the way he wanted. Now I'm scared he's going to die."

As you develop your care plan for Tom, you go about your normal tasks of coordinating transportation for him to get to dialysis, getting referrals for dialysis support groups, and coordinating information about his treatment with his primary physician. You are troubled, however, by Tom's refusal to look at lifestyle modification issues and by the stress his sister is experiencing.

1 Plan your search strategy ahead of time

2 Break down your search topic into components

You decide to go to the literature for information that can guide your management of this case. You need to find assessment tools to better evaluate Tom's psychological status. You suspect depression and alcoholism are present and are influencing Tom's behavior. Since it seems clear that Tom will not comply with any of the doctor's recommendations (stop smoking, stop drinking, follow diabetic diet, monitor blood glucose QID, reduce sodium intake, take medications), you want to learn about models of patient education. You also want to learn more about dealing with a patient's wishes, even when the patient seems to be self-destructive. Decide on the keywords, synonyms, or related terms of your search. The diagram below shows terms you should have considered. They have been grouped to make searching process easier.

What are the keywords, synonyms, or related terms?
- diabetes mellitus, insulin-dependent + education • patient education
- diabetes mellitus, insulin-dependent • patient compliance • self care

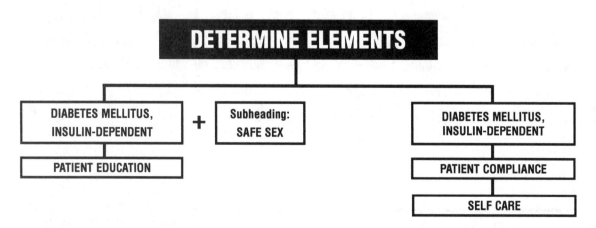

3 Check for subject headings in the Subject Heading List of the CINAHL® database

The following chart displays the subject headings exactly as they appear in the CINAHL Thesaurus.

THESAURUS

Subject Heading:
DIABETES MELLITUS, INSULIN-DEPENDENT

C18.452.297.267   C19.246.267
C20.111.327
Year: 1984
Diabetes mellitus characterized by insulin deficiency, sudden onset, severe hyperglycemia, rapid progression to ketoacidosis, and death unless treated with insulin. The disease may occur at any age, but onset occurs most commonly in childhood or adolescence.
see also INSULIN

x   Diabetes Mellitus, Juvenile Onset •
Diabetes Mellitus, Type 1 • IDDM •
Insulin-Dependent Diabetes Mellitus •
Juvenile Onset Diabetes Mellitus

Subject Heading:
PATIENT EDUCATION

I2.233.332.500+ $N2.421.143.824.407.680+
A combination of learning and motivation activities designed to educate patients and family members about disease states or procedures and appropriate methods for self-care. May occur in either inpatient or outpatient settings. Coordinate with specific disease or procedure/education. For articles that contain examples of patient education materials search for the document type "consumer/patient teaching materials."
see also KNOWLEDGE DEFICIT (NANDA) •
TEACHING: DISEASE PROCESS (IOWA NIC) •
TEACHING: GROUP (IOWA NIC) • TEACHING:
INDIVIDUAL (IOWA NIC) • TEACHING:
INFANT CARE (IOWA NIC) • TEACHING:
PRESCRIBED ACTIVITY/EXERCISE (IOWA
NIC) • TEACHING: PRESCRIBED DIET (IOWA
NIC)• TEACHING: PRESCRIBED MEDICATION
(IOWA NIC) • TEACHING: PSYCHOMOTOR
SKILL (IOWA NIC)

x   Education of Patients

Subheading:
EDUCATION or ED

Used for educating or teaching about diseases, procedures, services, or programs. Used for education and training in various disciplines and of various classes of people. Use available precoordinated education subject headings for formal educational programs. Use only for selected headings in the I2 tree. (C, E-N)

Subject Heading:
DIABETES MELLITUS, INSULIN-DEPENDENT

C18.452.297.267   C19.246.267
C20.111.327
Year: 1984
Diabetes mellitus characterized by insulin...

Subject Heading:
PATIENT COMPLIANCE

$F1.145.76.347.677 $F1.145.475.675
$F1.829.92.380.677 $F1.829.458.300.635
Voluntary cooperation of the patient in following a prescribed regimen.
see also EFFECTIVE MANAGEMENT OF
THERAPEUTIC REGIMEN: INDIVIDUAL
(NANDA) • NONCOMPLIANCE (NANDA)

x   Compliance, Patient • Patient
Cooperation • Regimen Adherence

XX   TREATMENT REFUSAL

Subject Heading:
SELF CARE

E2.900+
Consumer performance of activities for oneself traditionally performed by professional health care providers.
see also ACTIVITIES OF DAILY LIVING •
BATHING-HYGIENE SELF CARE DEFICIT
(NANDA) • DRESSING-GROOMING SELF
CARE DEFICIT (NANDA) • FEEDING SELF
CARE DEFICIT (NANDA) • OREM SELF-CARE
MODEL • SELF-CARE ASSISTANCE:
BATHING/HYGIENE (IOWA NIC) • SELF-CARE
ASSISTANCE: DRESSING/GROOMING (IOWA
NIC) • SELF-CARE ASSISTANCE: FEEDING
(IOWA NIC) • SELF-CARE ASSISTANCE
(IOWA NIC) • SELF-CARE ASSISTANCE:
TOILETING (IOWA NIC) • TOILETING SELF
CARE DEFICIT (NANDA)

x   Self Management

4 Decide which operators and limits you need

A OPERATORS

- Use operator "OR" to connect synonymous or related terms.
- Use operator "AND" to connect the different components – for example, *Diabetes Mellitus, Insulin-Dependent + education* AND *Patient Education*.

B LIMITS

- Limit your search by selecting the subheadings *education* when you search the subject heading *Diabetes Mellitus, Insulin-Dependent*.

C CONDUCTING YOUR SEARCHES

- You will be conducting your search using separate components and then combining these components to obtain the actual list of materials on your topic.

  1 The first group of terms you will search for is *Diabetes Mellitus, Insulin-Dependent + education – Patient Education*. When you search for the subject heading *Patient Education* select it and the specific terms under it by choosing the "explode" option.

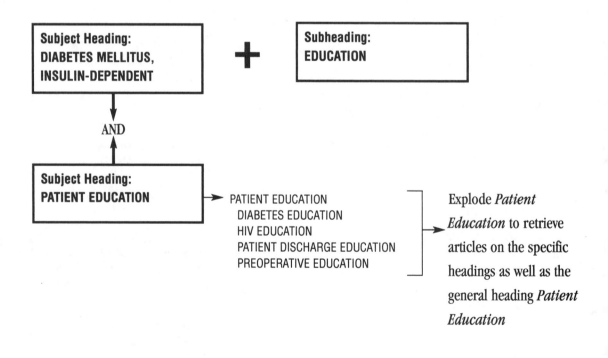

2 Then search for *Diabetes Mellitus, Insulin-Dependent + nursing – Patient Compliance – Self Care.* When you search for the subject heading *Self Care* select it and the specific terms under it by choosing the "explode" option.

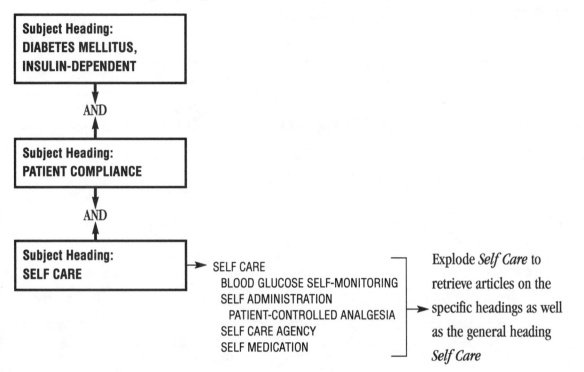

3 Finally, combine the components using the operator "OR".

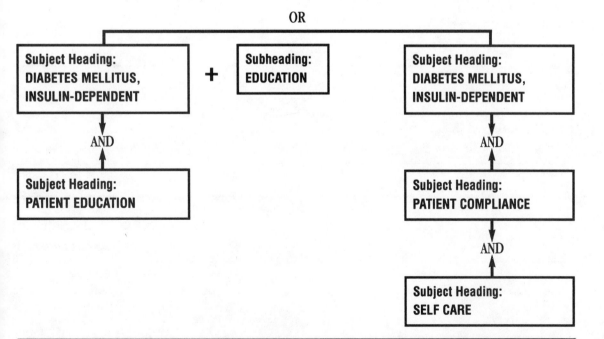

5   Run your search

6   View the results

NOTES

CASE STUDY 19

You are the nurse manager of obstetric services at your hospital. The policy in your labor and delivery unit (L&D) has been that no male health professional should be allowed to perform vaginal exams or other procedures involving the intimate exposure or touching of female patients unless a female health professional is also present as a chaperone. This has meant that all male obstetricians have had to have female nursing staff present during labor and delivery. This policy was implemented to protect the hospital and staff from potential lawsuits involving sexual misconduct toward its patients.

Until recently, this policy has never met any objections from doctors, nurses or patients. However, you have just received an application from a male nurse for an open position in L&D. The applicant has just moved to your city and appears to be well qualified. He has two years of experience in the normal birthing center and three years of experience on the high risk obstetrics unit of a major teaching hospital in the largest city in your region of the country. From his resume, he appears to have more education, specialized training, and experience than any of the other applicants.

Before you proceed with interviewing him, you need to deal with your unit's policy regarding unchaperoned male professionals. You know it would be impractical to require having a female nurse observe a male nurse every time he needed to perform a vaginal exam or do anything that might expose the patient. Having a male nurse would also complicate patient assignments, because, according to the policy, the male nurse could only be assigned to patients with female obstetricians. Otherwise, situations might arise where both the doctor and the nurse would be men and they would need to call in a third (female) staff person to chaperone them. You know that other units in your hospital do not carry chaperone restrictions on male nurses. They insert foley catheters, give baths, and toilet female patients without needing to be supervised. And there have never been any restrictions on female nurses doing procedures which involve the intimate exposure or touching of male patients.

1 Plan your search strategy ahead of time

2 Break down your search topic into components

Since the applicant seems to be so well qualified and comes with such excellent references, you decide to initiate a review of your unit's policy. Before you go to the administrators of the hospital, however, you need to do some research. You want to find out all you can about male nurses in labor and delivery. You need to find out if there have been any legal precedents either barring or permitting male nurses from working in obstetrics. What were the circumstances surrounding those decisions? Is your unit's policy similar to that of the hospitals involved in those legal cases? You also want to find out if male nurses in L&D are accepted by their patients and by the communities where those hospitals are located. Have the male L&D nurses been accepted by their female colleagues? Decide on the keywords, synonyms, or related terms of your search. The diagram below shows the terms you should have considered. They have been grouped together to make the searching process easier.

What are the keywords, synonyms, or related terms?

- students, nursing, male • nurses, male
- obstetric nursing • perinatal nursing

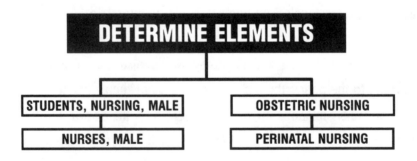

3 Check for subject headings in the Subject Heading List of the CINAHL® database

The following chart displays the subject headings exactly as they appear in the CINAHL Thesaurus.

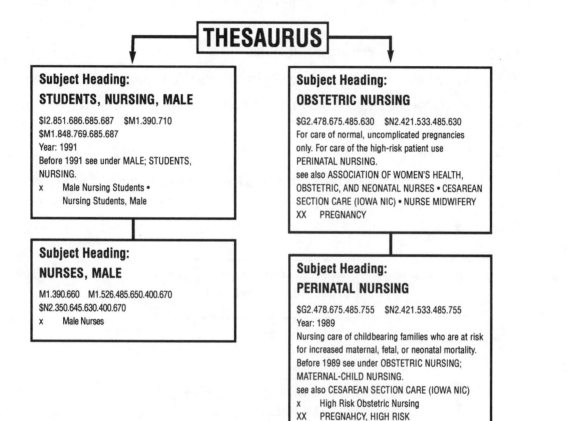

THESAURUS

Subject Heading:
STUDENTS, NURSING, MALE

$I2.851.686.685.687 $M1.390.710
$M1.848.769.685.687
Year: 1991
Before 1991 see under MALE; STUDENTS, NURSING.
x   Male Nursing Students •
    Nursing Students, Male

Subject Heading:
NURSES, MALE

M1.390.660   M1.526.485.650.400.670
$N2.350.645.630.400.670
x   Male Nurses

Subject Heading:
OBSTETRIC NURSING

$G2.478.675.485.630 $N2.421.533.485.630
For care of normal, uncomplicated pregnancies
only. For care of the high-risk patient use
PERINATAL NURSING.
see also ASSOCIATION OF WOMEN'S HEALTH,
OBSTETRIC, AND NEONATAL NURSES • CESAREAN
SECTION CARE (IOWA NIC) • NURSE MIDWIFERY
XX   PREGNANCY

Subject Heading:
PERINATAL NURSING

$G2.478.675.485.755 $N2.421.533.485.755
Year: 1989
Nursing care of childbearing families who are at risk
for increased maternal, fetal, or neonatal mortality.
Before 1989 see under OBSTETRIC NURSING;
MATERNAL-CHILD NURSING.
see also CESAREAN SECTION CARE (IOWA NIC)
x   High Risk Obstetric Nursing
XX   PREGNAHCY, HIGH RISK

4 Decide which operators you need

A OPERATORS

- Use operator "OR" to connect synonymous or related terms – for example, *Students, Nursing, Male* OR *Nurses, Male*.

- Use operator "AND" to connect the different components.

B CONDUCTING YOUR SEARCHES

- You will be conducting your search using separate components and then combining these components to obtain the actual list of materials on your topic.

    1   The first group of terms you will search for is *Students, Nursing, Male – Nurses, Male*.

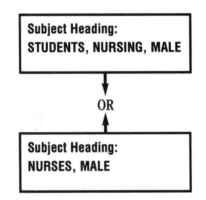

2 The second group of terms you will search for is *Obstetric Nursing – Perinatal Nursing*.

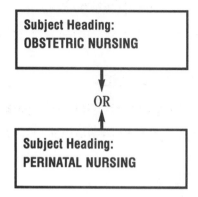

3 Finally, combine the components using the operator "AND".

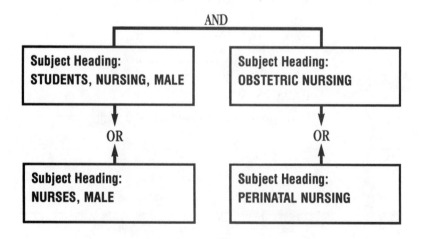

5   Run your search

6   View the results

NOTES

CASE STUDY 20

You are a school nurse working in the student health center. A student comes in with bruises to his face, a cut lip, and ripped clothes. While you treat his injuries, you try to find out what happened. You learn that Michael, age 16, was cornered by a group of guys who beat him up while yelling derogatory names at him. "They kept pushing and hitting me, shouting things like 'We don't want fags in our school,' and 'All queers should die.'" Michael was shaken up badly by this attack and wonders aloud whether it might be safer for him to drop out of school.

Because of the psychological trauma Michael experienced, you spend additional time with him to offer counseling and support. Michael describes himself as never having fit in with the guys at school and frequently being called a "sissy." He says that since he doesn't have many friends, he studies a lot and that he has always been a straight "A" student. After developing some rapport with Michael, he tells you that he has recently accepted that he is gay. "It's something I've always known about myself, I just didn't want to admit it. And now that I've started to 'come out', I get beat up."

You ask him whether "coming out" means he has become sexually active, to which he responds affirmatively. You ask him questions regarding his knowledge of HIV and safer sex guidelines. Michael's responds that "AIDS is something only gay men in places like New York and San Francisco get," and that since he lives in a smaller city he doesn't need to worry about it. You also assess whether his family is supportive, or whether he has any gay friends. He tells you that if his family found out they'd disown him, and that he doesn't know anyone else in school who is gay. "Since I look older than I am, I can get into the gay bar in town. That's where I've started to hang out and meet other gay men."

You realize that Michael is at high risk for many problems: further violence from his classmates, dropping out of school even though he is an excellent student, contracting HIV or other sexually transmitted diseases, developing an alcohol or drug problem related to using these substances (at the gay bar) at a vulnerable developmental stage, and for other emotional problems related to lack of family support or friends. During your time with Michael you give him information about HIV and safe sex, but realize that all your literature on STDs is geared towards young heterosexual clients and is not really appropriate for gay teens. You ask Michael whether he would like having your office be a "safe place" for him to drop by to talk about what's happening in his life, and he agrees.

1 Plan your search strategy ahead of time

2 Break down your search topic into components

Your work is cut out for you. You need to go to the literature to find information on homosexuality and teenagers. You want to learn more about the experience of gay teens, as well as how you as a health professional can contribute to their physical and psychological well being. You know statistically that Michael cannot be the only gay person in your school. Perhaps there is something in the literature that describes how to start a support group for students who might be questioning their sexual orientation. This beating incident makes you realize that students in your school need to learn more about homosexuality, homophobia, and learning to deal with differences. You are hoping that the literature can give you ideas for introducing these topics into your school so that all students can feel safe. Decide on the keywords, synonyms, or related terms of your search. The diagram below shows terms you should have considered. They have been grouped to make the searching process easier.

What are the keywords, synonyms, or related terms?
- homosexuality • homosexuals, male • homophobia

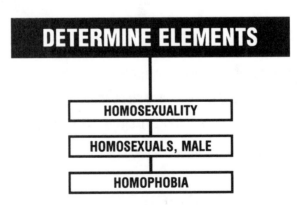

DETERMINE ELEMENTS

| HOMOSEXUALITY |
| HOMOSEXUALS, MALE |
| HOMOPHOBIA |

3 Check for subject headings in the Subject Heading List of the CINAHL® database

The following chart displays the subject headings exactly as they appear in the CINAHL Thesaurus.

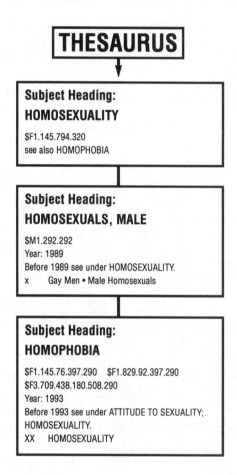

THESAURUS

Subject Heading:
HOMOSEXUALITY

$F1.145.794.320
see also HOMOPHOBIA

Subject Heading:
HOMOSEXUALS, MALE

$M1.292.292
Year: 1989
Before 1989 see under HOMOSEXUALITY.
x   Gay Men • Male Homosexuals

Subject Heading:
HOMOPHOBIA

$F1.145.76.397.290 $F1.829.92.397.290
$F3.709.438.180.508.290
Year: 1993
Before 1993 see under ATTITUDE TO SEXUALITY;
HOMOSEXUALITY.
XX   HOMOSEXUALITY

4 Decide which operators and limits you need

A OPERATORS

- Use operator "OR" to connect synonymous or related terms – for example, *Homosexuality* OR *Homosexuals, Male* OR *Homophobia*.

B LIMITS

- Limit your search by using the population group *adolescence*.

C CONDUCTING YOUR SEARCHES

- You will be conducting your search using separate components and then combining these components to obtain the actual list of materials on your topic.

- You will search for the terms *Homosexuality – Homosexuals, Male – Homophobia* and limit your search using the population group *adolescence*.

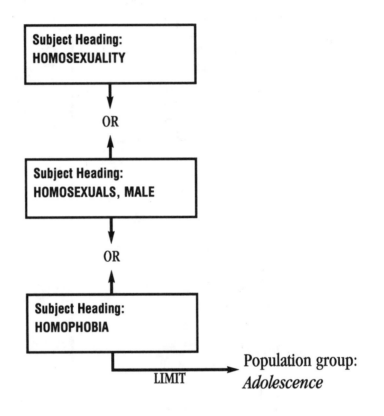

5   Run your search

6   View the results

NOTES

CASE STUDY 21

You are a veteran nurse with 16 years of experience. You originally got your RN license after attending a diploma program. After ten years of working in several different hospitals in medical-surgical units, ICU, and the emergency room, you went back to school to get your BSN degree. You have continued to work in the acute care setting. Although you have considered moving into management, you realize that your primary interest is in providing direct patient care. Therefore, you have continued in your position as charge nurse for the medical-surgical unit at your hospital.

During your years of work you have seen nursing, and the healthcare field in general, undergo many changes. You have experienced changes in staffing patterns which utilize various skill mixes of nurses and assistants with different levels of training. You have seen changes in medical procedures which have affected the types of patients you see and the length of time they are in the hospital. Most recently you have seen the effect that managed care is having on the healthcare system. One hospital in your city recently closed after it lost its bid for a contract with the major managed care insurer in your region. Your own hospital is rumored to be considering merging with another hospital in your area. Nurses everywhere, even those with years of experience, are being told to prepare for layoffs.

1 Plan your search strategy ahead of time

2 Break down your search topic into components

You have been considering going back to school to get an MSN degree. Before you make your decision, however, you want to learn more about the direction the nursing profession is going. You want to learn more about the way in which the healthcare system is being reorganized and how this is related to the hospital closures and mergers that seem to be happening everywhere. You know you need to learn more about the economic realities of healthcare delivery and want to know what role nursing plays in this larger picture. And of course, you want to learn more about your own prospects for employment in the future. From what you find, you hope to be able to make your decision about whether to pursue an additional nursing degree. Although your interest in graduate work is partly tied to your desire for personal growth, you are also pragmatic and want to know whether additional schooling will add to your job security. While you are committed to direct patient care as your career, you also are interested in how pursuing an advanced degree can help secure the role of nursing in the changing healthcare environment. You decide to search the nursing literature for information that will address these issues. Decide on the keywords, synonyms, or related terms of your search. The diagram below shows terms you should have considered. They have been grouped to make the searching process easier.

What are the keywords, synonyms, or related terms?

- nursing as a profession + trends • nursing role • nursing practice + trends
- health care delivery + economics
- education, nursing, graduate • masters-prepared nurses
- employment

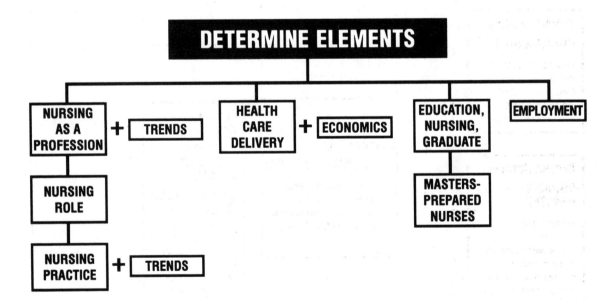

3 Check for subject headings in the Subject Heading List of the CINAHL® database

The following chart displays the subject headings exactly as they appear in the CINAHL Thesaurus.

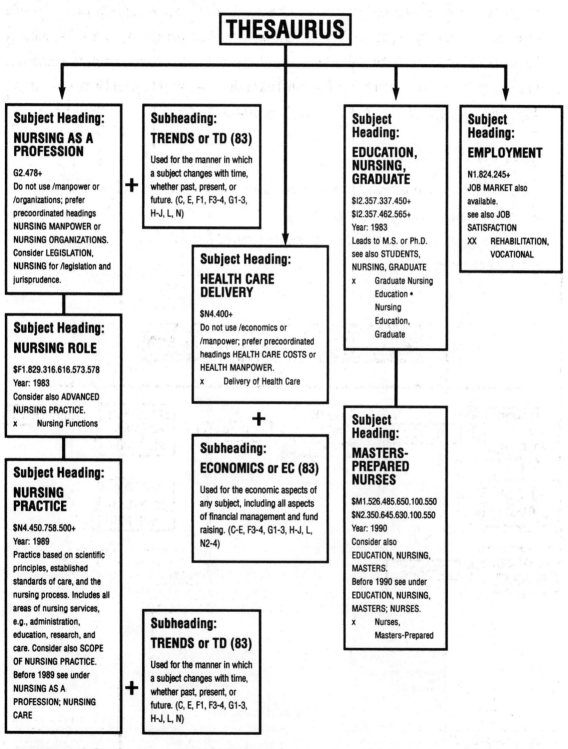

THESAURUS

Subject Heading:
NURSING AS A PROFESSION

G2.478+
Do not use /manpower or /organizations; prefer precoordinated headings NURSING MANPOWER or NURSING ORGANIZATIONS. Consider LEGISLATION, NURSING for /legislation and jurisprudence.

Subheading:
TRENDS or TD (83)

Used for the manner in which a subject changes with time, whether past, present, or future. (C, E, F1, F3-4, G1-3, H-J, L, N)

Subject Heading:
EDUCATION, NURSING, GRADUATE

$12.357.337.450+
$12.357.462.565+
Year: 1983
Leads to M.S. or Ph.D.
see also STUDENTS, NURSING, GRADUATE
x   Graduate Nursing Education •
     Nursing Education, Graduate

Subject Heading:
EMPLOYMENT

N1.824.245+
JOB MARKET also available.
see also JOB SATISFACTION
XX   REHABILITATION, VOCATIONAL

Subject Heading:
NURSING ROLE

$F1.829.316.616.573.578
Year: 1983
Consider also ADVANCED NURSING PRACTICE.
x   Nursing Functions

Subject Heading:
HEALTH CARE DELIVERY

$N4.400+
Do not use /economics or /manpower; prefer precoordinated headings HEALTH CARE COSTS or HEALTH MANPOWER.
x   Delivery of Health Care

Subject Heading:
NURSING PRACTICE

$N4.450.758.500+
Year: 1989
Practice based on scientific principles, established standards of care, and the nursing process. Includes all areas of nursing services, e.g., administration, education, research, and care. Consider also SCOPE OF NURSING PRACTICE. Before 1989 see under NURSING AS A PROFESSION; NURSING CARE

Subheading:
ECONOMICS or EC (83)

Used for the economic aspects of any subject, including all aspects of financial management and fund raising. (C-E, F3-4, G1-3, H-J, L, N2-4)

Subject Heading:
MASTERS-PREPARED NURSES

$M1.526.485.650.100.550
$N2.350.645.630.100.550
Year: 1990
Consider also EDUCATION, NURSING, MASTERS.
Before 1990 see under EDUCATION, NURSING, MASTERS; NURSES.
x   Nurses, Masters-Prepared

Subheading:
TRENDS or TD (83)

Used for the manner in which a subject changes with time, whether past, present, or future. (C, E, F1, F3-4, G1-3, H-J, L, N)

4 Decide which operators and limits you need

A OPERATORS

- Use operator "OR" to connect synonymous or related terms – for example, *Education, Nursing, Graduate* OR *Masters-Prepared Nurses*.
- Use operator "AND" to connect the different components.

B LIMITS

- **Subheadings**. Limit your search using subheadings as follows:

  Nursing as a Profession + trends

  Health Care Delivery + economics

  Nursing Practice + trends

C CONDUCTING YOUR SEARCHES

- You will be conducting your search using separate components and then combining these components to obtain the actual list of materials on your topic.

1 The first group of terms you will search for is *Nursing as a Profession + trends – Nursing Role – Nursing Practice + trends*. Limit *Nursing as a Profession* and *Nursing Practice* by selecting the subheading *trends*.

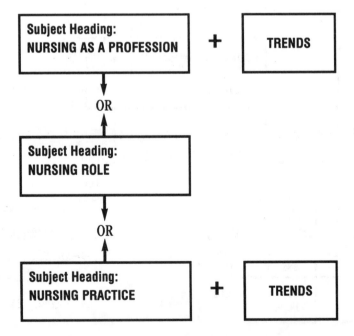

2 The next term you will search for is *Health Care Delivery*. Select it and the specific terms under it by choosing the "explode" option. Limit using the subheading *economics*.

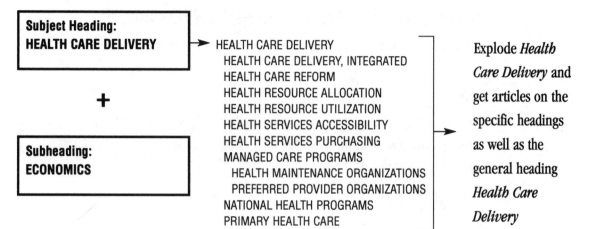

Subject Heading:
HEALTH CARE DELIVERY

+

Subheading:
ECONOMICS

HEALTH CARE DELIVERY
  HEALTH CARE DELIVERY, INTEGRATED
  HEALTH CARE REFORM
  HEALTH RESOURCE ALLOCATION
  HEALTH RESOURCE UTILIZATION
  HEALTH SERVICES ACCESSIBILITY
  HEALTH SERVICES PURCHASING
  MANAGED CARE PROGRAMS
    HEALTH MAINTENANCE ORGANIZATIONS
    PREFERRED PROVIDER ORGANIZATIONS
  NATIONAL HEALTH PROGRAMS
  PRIMARY HEALTH CARE

Explode *Health Care Delivery* and get articles on the specific headings as well as the general heading *Health Care Delivery*

3 The third group of terms you will search for is *Education, Nursing, Graduate – Masters-Prepared Nurses*.

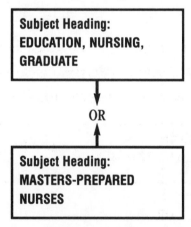

Subject Heading:
EDUCATION, NURSING, GRADUATE

OR

Subject Heading:
MASTERS-PREPARED NURSES

4 Next search for the term *Employment*. Select it and the specific terms under it by choosing the "explode" option.

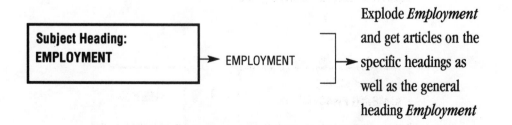

Subject Heading:
EMPLOYMENT

EMPLOYMENT

Explode *Employment* and get articles on the specific headings as well as the general heading *Employment*

5 Finally, combine the components using operators: [(*Nursing as a Profession + trends* OR *Nursing Role* OR *Nursing Practice + trends*) AND (*Health Care Delivery + economics*)] OR [(*Education, Nursing, Graduate* OR *Masters-Prepared Nurses*) AND (*Employment*)].

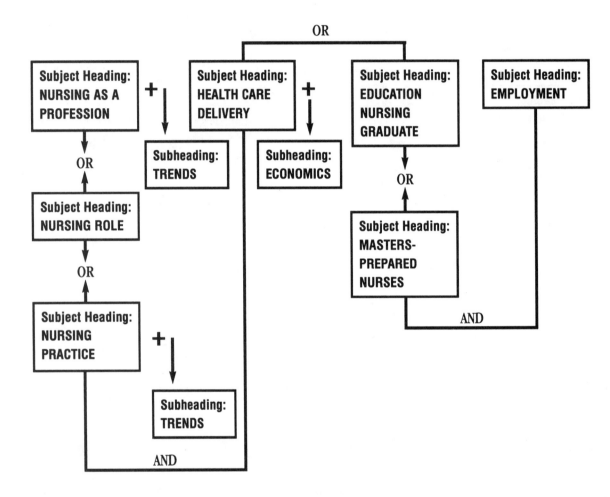

5   Run your search

6   View the results

NOTES

CASE STUDY 22

You are the director of a nursing program at a state university. Your graduates receive a BSN and are prepared to take the RN licensing examination. With the many changes in the healthcare delivery system, however, you are having to consider restructuring your program. Reduced hospital lengths of stay have resulted in such low hospital census that there are often not enough patients for your students to gain solid clinical experience during their various rotations (medical-surgical, maternity, pediatrics, and psychiatric nursing). Upon graduation, your students are having a hard time finding jobs. Hospitals everywhere have fewer inpatients and are responding by laying off even experienced nurses. Those hospitals which are hiring nurses can demand that applicants have experience.

The move in healthcare has been to shift delivery of services as soon as possible from the acute care setting to patients' homes. In order to adapt your nursing program to this change, you want to develop a special emphasis in your curriculum on nursing care in the community/home setting. By doing this, you hope your curriculum will more adequately prepare them for providing care in settings where most of them will eventually work. You also hope to give your students practical experience that will help them in their initial search for jobs in the community after graduation.

1 Plan your search strategy ahead of time

2 Break down your search topic into components

As you design the new curriculum, you decide to search the literature to see what other nursing schools are doing to address the impact changes in healthcare are having on nursing. You hope to find references to other nursing programs that have an emphasis on nursing care in the community/home setting. Because the success of the changes you hope to implement will depend on collaboration with many community health agencies, you also want to find references on developing partnerships between educational institutions and service providers in the community. Decide on the keywords, synonyms, or related terms of your search. The diagram below shows terms you should have considered. They have been grouped to make the searching process easier.

What are the keywords, synonyms, or related terms?

- community health nursing • home nursing, professional
- curriculum
- education, nursing
- collaboration

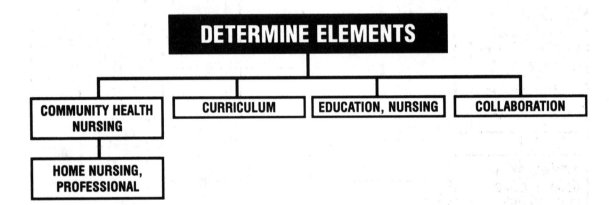

3 Check for subject headings in the Subject Heading List of the CINAHL® database

The following chart displays the subject headings exactly as they appear in the CINAHL Thesaurus.

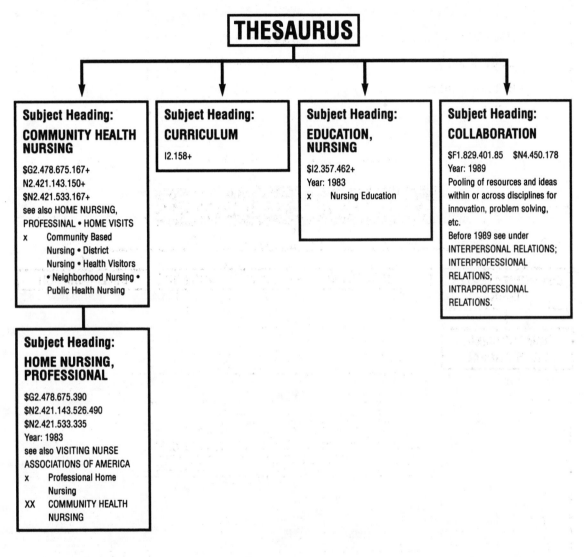

THESAURUS

Subject Heading:
COMMUNITY HEALTH NURSING

$G2.478.675.167+
N2.421.143.150+
$N2.421.533.167+
see also HOME NURSING, PROFESSIONAL • HOME VISITS
x   Community Based Nursing • District Nursing • Health Visitors • Neighborhood Nursing • Public Health Nursing

Subject Heading:
CURRICULUM

I2.158+

Subject Heading:
EDUCATION, NURSING

$I2.357.462+
Year: 1983
x   Nursing Education

Subject Heading:
COLLABORATION

$F1.829.401.85 $N4.450.178
Year: 1989
Pooling of resources and ideas within or across disciplines for innovation, problem solving, etc.
Before 1989 see under INTERPERSONAL RELATIONS; INTERPROFESSIONAL RELATIONS; INTRAPROFESSIONAL RELATIONS.

Subject Heading:
HOME NURSING, PROFESSIONAL

$G2.478.675.390
$N2.421.143.526.490
$N2.421.533.335
Year: 1983
see also VISITING NURSE ASSOCIATIONS OF AMERICA
x   Professional Home Nursing
XX   COMMUNITY HEALTH NURSING

4 Decide which operators and limits you need

A OPERATORS

- Use operator "OR" to connect synonymous or related terms – for example, *Community Health Nursing* OR *Home Nursing, Professional*.

- Use operator "AND" to connect the different components.

B LIMITS

- **Major focus**. Choose to modify ALL the subject headings by selecting materials that focus on the topics (major subject headings).

C CONDUCTING YOUR SEARCHES

- You will be conducting your search using separate components and then combining these components to obtain the actual list of materials on your topic.

    1 The first group of terms you will search for is *Community Health Nursing – Home Nursing, Professional*.

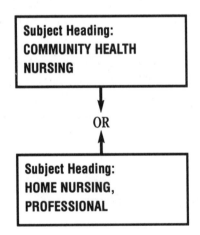

2 Next search for *Curriculum.* Select it and the specific terms under it by choosing the "explode" option.

```
┌─────────────────────────┐
│ Subject Heading:        │
│ CURRICULUM              │──────▶   CURRICULUM ──────────────┐      Explode *Curriculum*
│                         │            COURSE CONTENT         │      and get articles on the
└─────────────────────────┘            COURSE EVALUATION      │──▶   specific headings as
                                        CURRICULUM DEVELOPMENT │      well as the general
                                        INTEGRATED CURRICULUM ─┘      heading *Curriculum*
```

3 Then search for *Education, Nursing.* When you choose this subject heading select it and the specific terms under it by choosing the "explode" option.

```
┌─────────────────────────┐
│ Subject Heading:        │
│ EDUCATION, NURSING      │──────▶  EDUCATION, NURSING ──────────────────┐    Explode
│                         │           EDUCATION, NURSE ANESTHESIA        │    *Education,*
└─────────────────────────┘           EDUCATION, NURSE MIDWIFERY         │    *Nursing* and
                                       EDUCATION, NURSING, ASSOCIATE      │    get articles on
                                       EDUCATION, NURSING, BACCALAUREATE  │    the specific
                                         EDUCATION, POST-RN               │──▶ headings as
                                       EDUCATION, NURSING, CONTINUING     │    well as the
                                       EDUCATION, NURSING, DIPLOMA PROGRAMS│   general
                                       EDUCATION, NURSING, GRADUATE       │    heading
                                         EDUCATION, NURSING DOCTORAL      │    *Education,*
                                         EDUCATION, NURSING, MASTERS      │    *Nursing*
                                         EDUCATION, NURSING, POST-DOCTORAL│
                                       EDUCATION, NURSING, PRACTICAL      │
                                       EDUCATION, NURSING, RESEARCH BASED ┘
```

4 Next search for *Collaboration.*

```
        ┌─────────────────────────┐
        │ Subject Heading:        │
        │ COLLABORATION           │
        └─────────────────────────┘
```

5 Finally, combine the components using the operators: (*Community Health Nursing* OR *Home Nursing, Professional*) AND (*Curriculum* OR *Education, Nursing*) OR (*Education, Nursing* AND *Collaboration*).

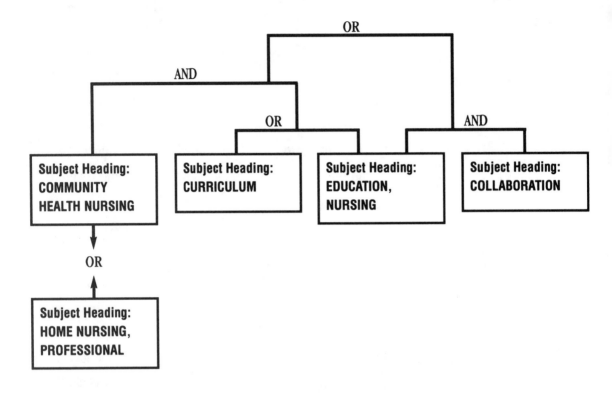

5   Run your search

6   View the results

NOTES

CASE STUDY 23

You are a nurse working through a community agency which provides follow-up home visits to patients who have been in the hospital. Harry is a 70-year-old man who had a myocardial infarction (MI), followed by a triple coronary artery bypass graft (CABG). Harry is six weeks post-op and his doctor has ordered visits by a nurse to begin a home exercise program to increase his activity tolerance. From your knowledge of coronary artery disease, you know that you will also be assessing Harry for other risk factors related to heart disease, such as smoking, stress, and a diet high in fats and cholesterol.

During your initial visit, you find Harry's sternal incision is well healed and that he has not experienced any episodes of angina since the operation. He states, however, that he has so little energy that he can hardly get out of bed in the morning. You explain that the purpose of your visits is to help him get more energy so that he can resume his normal activities. He is receptive and agrees to follow the exercise plan you propose. The first session you show him how to do chair exercises while sitting. This mild activity raises his pulse from 72 bpm to 80 bpm. You determine that this is a safe level of activity to begin his program. You confirm that he knows how to take his pulse and instruct him to do this set of exercises every day for the next week.

At your second visit you assess Harry's other cardiovascular risk factors. You find out that Harry quit smoking 20 years ago and that he changed his diet to a low-fat, low-cholesterol diet five years ago when he was first diagnosed with CAD. He admits that he feels a lot of stress in his life. His wife of 45 years had a stroke last year which left her paralyzed on one side and is in a nursing home. He is estranged from his three children who all live far away. He says he used to deal with his stress by going on fishing trips, but he doubts if he'll ever be able to do that again. You ask him how he did with his exercises during the past week. He says he did them three days out of the last week, but the other days he felt too "stressed out" to muster up the strength.

As you continue to increase Harry's exercise program to standing exercises, then walking around the house and then walking up and down the block, you note Harry expresses little emotion and always has a flat affect. Although he has been able to comply with his exercise regime enough to continue increasing the duration and intensity, his self-report is that he is only doing his exercise program about half the time. He frequently talks about feeling too "stressed out" to do more, even though he admits the exercise makes him feel better. You begin to suspect that Harry is actually suffering from depression and that he is using references to stress as a way of talking about it.

1 Plan your search strategy ahead of time

2 Break down your search topic into components

You decide to search the literature for books and journal articles about depression in the elderly. You want to find out more about the unique ways in which depression presents itself among elderly persons and whether it is treated differently when the person is elderly. Because of Harry's avoidance of the term "depression" you want to learn more about the stigma people of his generation may feel about mental illness. You wonder whether there are interventions you can use to move him toward recognizing his need for help without making him feel stigmatized. You are concerned that, if untreated, Harry's depression will interfere with his long-term compliance with his exercise program which could impact his risk of future cardiac events. Decide on the keywords, synonyms, or related terms of your search. The diagram below shows the terms you should have considered. They have been grouped to make the searching process easier.

What are the keywords, synonyms, or related terms?

- coronary disease • cardiac patients • rehabilitation, cardiac
- depression • psychosocial aspects of illness

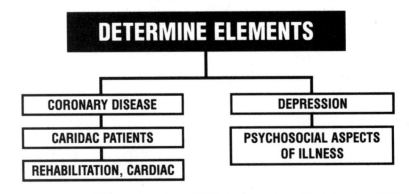

3 Check for subject headings in the Subject Heading List of the CINAHL® database

The following chart displays the subject headings exactly as they appear in the CINAHL Thesaurus.

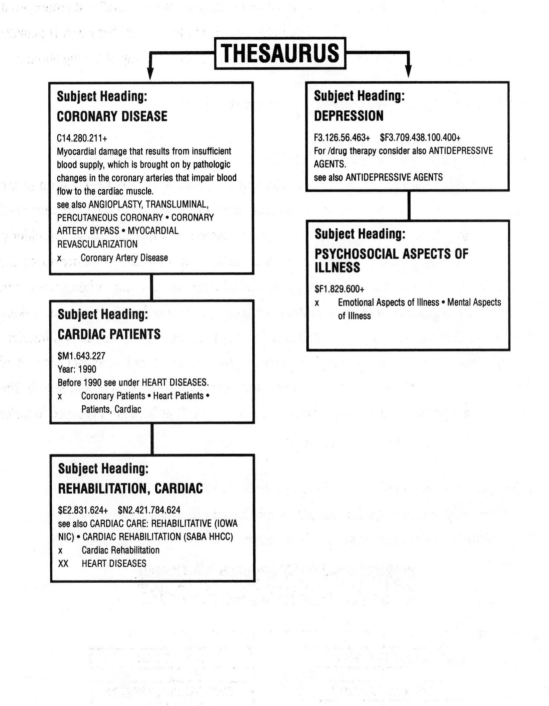

THESAURUS

Subject Heading:
CORONARY DISEASE

C14.280.211+
Myocardial damage that results from insufficient blood supply, which is brought on by pathologic changes in the coronary arteries that impair blood flow to the cardiac muscle.
see also ANGIOPLASTY, TRANSLUMINAL, PERCUTANEOUS CORONARY • CORONARY ARTERY BYPASS • MYOCARDIAL REVASCULARIZATION
x   Coronary Artery Disease

Subject Heading:
CARDIAC PATIENTS

$M1.643.227
Year: 1990
Before 1990 see under HEART DISEASES.
x   Coronary Patients • Heart Patients • Patients, Cardiac

Subject Heading:
REHABILITATION, CARDIAC

$E2.831.624+ $N2.421.784.624
see also CARDIAC CARE: REHABILITATIVE (IOWA NIC) • CARDIAC REHABILITATION (SABA HHCC)
x   Cardiac Rehabilitation
XX   HEART DISEASES

Subject Heading:
DEPRESSION

F3.126.56.463+ $F3.709.438.100.400+
For /drug therapy consider also ANTIDEPRESSIVE AGENTS.
see also ANTIDEPRESSIVE AGENTS

Subject Heading:
PSYCHOSOCIAL ASPECTS OF ILLNESS

$F1.829.600+
x   Emotional Aspects of Illness • Mental Aspects of Illness

4 Decide which operators and limits you need

A OPERATORS

- Use operator "OR" to connect synonymous or related terms – for example, *Depression* OR *Psychosocial Aspects of Illness*.
- Use operator "AND" to connect the different components.

B LIMITS

- Limit your search using the limits *aged* and *male*.

C CONDUCTING YOUR SEARCHES

- You will be conducting your search using separate components and then combining these components to obtain the actual list of materials on your topic.

  1 The first group of terms you will search for is *Coronary Disease – Cardiac Patients – Rehabilitation, Cardiac*. When you search for *Coronary Disease* and *Rehabilitation, Cardiac* select them and the specific terms under them by choosing the "explode" option.

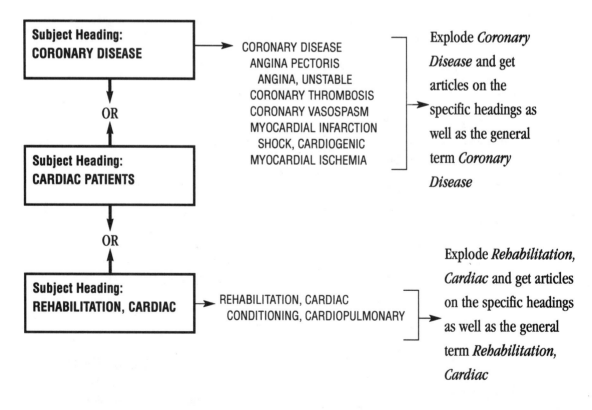

2 The second group of terms you will search for is *depression –*
psychosocial aspects of illness. Select it and the specific terms under it by
choosing the "explode" option.

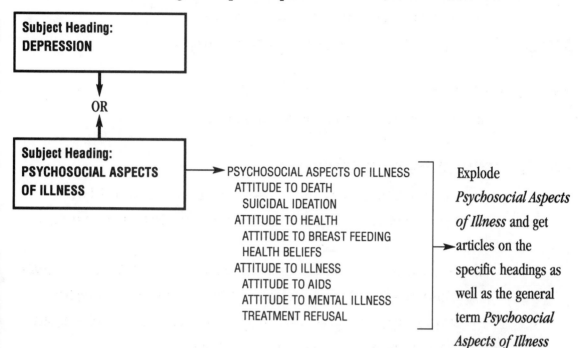

3 Finally, combine the components using the operator "OR" and limit your
search using the population groups *aged* and *male*.

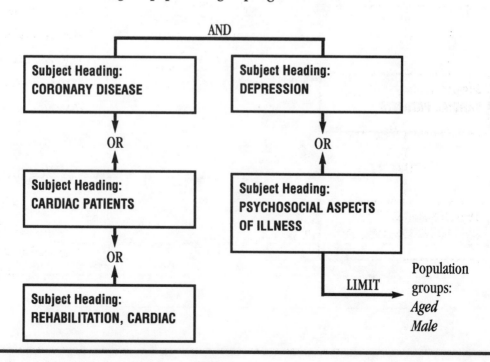

5   Run your search

6   View the results

NOTES

CASE STUDY 24

You are a public health nurse in a rural area. Half of your job is spent making home visits to people across a three-county area. The other half of your job is to direct educational campaigns around issues that affect public health. One of the main issues that concerns you is smoking and the health effects it is having on your clients.

Sixty-five percent of men and 50% of women over 18 in your area are smokers. This is more than double the national smoking rate. It is not surprising, therefore, that deaths in your counties due to heart disease, cancer, and chronic respiratory conditions are much higher than seen nationally. The hospitals in your counties also report having a disproportionally large number of low birth weight babies. The majority of your home visits are to provide follow-up care for smoking related illnesses. Most people in your area start smoking when they are in high school. By the time kids graduate from high school, almost 80% of them smoke on a daily basis. Thus, they enter adulthood solidly addicted to nicotine.

1 Plan your search strategy ahead of time

2 Break down your search topic into components

You want to develop a multi-pronged community education program to reduce the rate of smoking across all age groups. You decide to search the literature to find out what kinds of programs have been successfully implemented in other communities. You are interested in those that target youth as well as adults. You are particularly interested in finding out about community education programs that have been implemented in rural areas. You know that you will need to collaborate with schools, churches, businesses, and other community agencies, and hope to find in the literature references on how to build community coalitions to get broad-based support for your program. You also want to find guidelines for how to construct the evaluation component of this type of community education program so that you will be able to establish the effectiveness of your work. Decide on the keywords, synonyms, or related terms of your search. The diagram below shows the terms you should have considered. They have been grouped to make the searching process easier.

What are the keywords, synonyms, or related terms?
- smoking + prevention and control • smoking cessation programs
- community health services • community health nursing

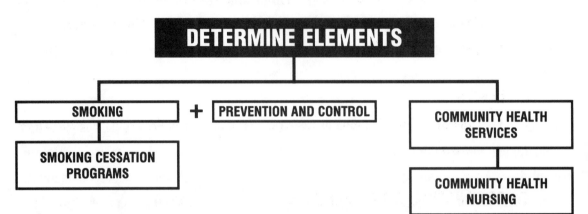

3 Check for subject headings in the Subject Heading List of the CINAHL® database

The following chart displays the subject headings exactly as they appear in the CINAHL Thesaurus.

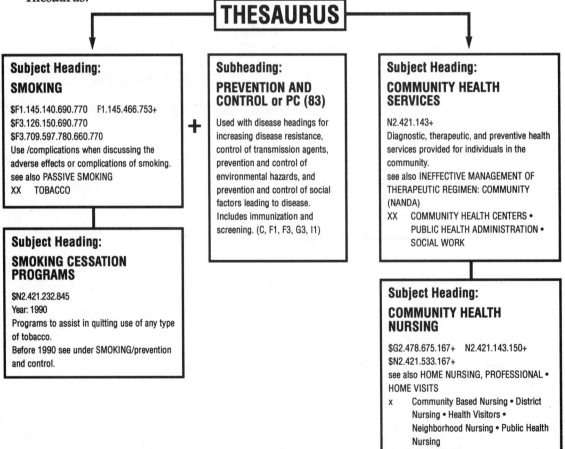

4 Decide which operators and limits you need

A OPERATORS

- Use operator "OR" to connect synonymous or related terms – for example, *Smoking + prevention and control* OR *Smoking Cessation Programs*.
- Use operator "AND" to connect the different components.

B LIMITS

- Limit the subject heading *Smoking* by selecting the subheading *prevention and control*.

C CONDUCTING YOUR SEARCHES

- You will be conducting your search using separate components and then combining these components to obtain the actual list of materials on your topic.

  1 The first group of terms you will search for is *Smoking + prevention and control – Smoking Cessation Programs*.

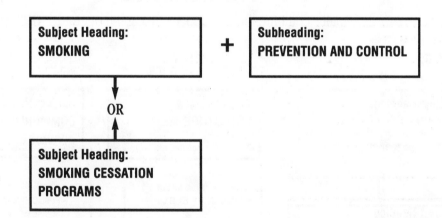

2 The second group of terms you will search for will be *Community Health Services – Community Health Nursing*. When you search the subject heading *Community Health Services* select it and the specific terms under it by choosing the "explode" option.

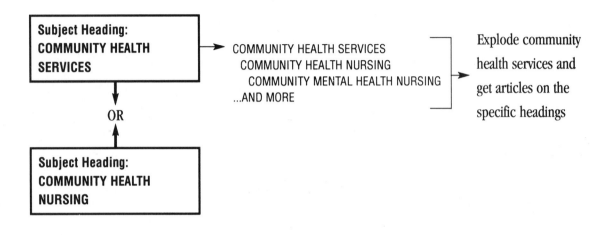

3 Finally, combine the components using the operator "OR".

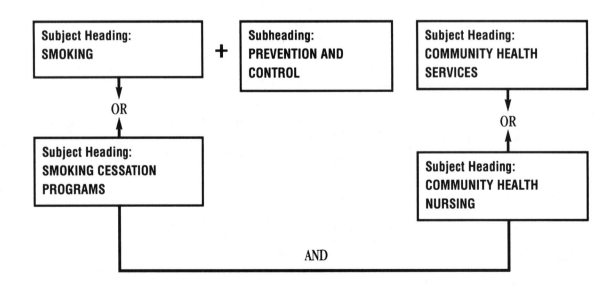

5   Run your search

6   View the results

NOTES

Appendix 1

SELECTING THE APPROPRIATE DATABASE

What subjects are covered in the search and which bibliographic database focuses on those subject areas specifically?

A thorough knowledge of the subject coverage of a database ensures the most informed database selection decisions. It is not only important to know what subjects are covered, but also those which are excluded. For example, the CINAHL® database has a strong nursing and allied health orientation, plus access to biomedicine and consumer health information and the library literature. Virtually all English-language and selected non-English nursing journals are indexed along with journals in 17 allied health disciplines. The 17 disciplines are cardiopulmonary technology, dental hygiene, emergency services, medical/laboratory technology, the medical assistant, medical records, nutrition and dietetics, occupational therapy, optometry, physical therapy and rehabilitation, the physician's assistant, podiatry, radiologic technology, respiratory therapy, social service in health care, speech-language pathology and audiology, and surgical technology. In 1988 journals in health sciences librarianship were included. Consumer health was added in 1991. Selective coverage is also provided for journals in the behavioral sciences, management, education, and alternative therapies.

What type of resource contains material on the subject and what database covers the format required?

The CINAHL database covers journal articles, books and book chapters, pamphlets and pamphlet chapters, dissertations, standards of professional practice, conference proceedings, educational software, audiovisuals, nurse practice acts, critical paths, research instruments, legal cases, accreditation records, and clinical innovation records.

Does the database cover the years required?

The CINAHL database includes indexing from January 1982 to the present.

How often is the database updated?

The CINAHL database is updated monthly.

What is the size of the database?

As of June 1998, the CINAHL database contained 382,248 records. In total, over 1,100 journals are regularly scanned and indexed.

Are journals indexed on a cover-to-cover basis or are only selected references added?

Nursing and allied health journals are indexed cover-to-cover, while the rest of the journals are selectively indexed in the CINAHL® database.

How heavily may a searcher rely on the Subject Heading List of a database?

Specific and current subject headings that accurately reflect the nursing and allied health literature are established on an ongoing basis. However, new headings are added to the thesaurus only once a year. New terms assigned to material in the database during the year can only be searched as keywords in the terms in process field.

The CINAHL Subject Heading List (Thesaurus) is updated annually. If appropriate, one-for-one changes from the old subject headings to new terms are made at the same time. The CINAHL Subject Heading List includes more than 2,500 unique headings for specific concepts in nursing and allied health. Vocabulary covering the nursing specialties, nursing theorists, NANDA nursing diagnoses terms, etc., have been added to facilitate easy access to the nursing literature. MeSH headings are used for disease, physiology, and drug terms.

What kind of indexing is provided by the database? Is it specific and in-depth or is broader coverage provided?

CINAHL indexers work hard to establish logical and consistent guidelines for indexing. Specific and current subject headings that accurately reflect nursing and allied health literature are established. In order to correctly assign these headings the indexers refer to thesaurus scope notes, cross-references, and tree structures.

Complex subjects are indexed following a series of guidelines, listed here in order of preference:

1 Precoordinated main headings for commonly occurring concepts, e.g., *Lung* and *Neoplasms = Lung Neoplasms*
2 Main headings/subheading combination e.g., *Schools, Nursing/evaluation*
3 Main heading plus document type, e.g., *Psychiatric Nursing* (care plan)
4 Main heading plus population group, e.g., *Breast Neoplasms*-female
5 Two or more main headings, e.g., *Home Childbirth; Midwifery*

The indexers assign the most specific headings available. The indexers assign as many items as are necessary to cover the content fully. The terms are assigned as either major or minor descriptors.

The nursing and allied health journal are indexed in-depth, while books, book chapters, software, audiovisuals, and consumer health material are indexed less in-depth.

Which database allows you to find answers to specific questions?

Subject headings, no matter how reliable, cannot always answer all information needs. The CINAHL® database has many other access points that can help in almost any situation, such as title, series title, abstract, author's name, accession numbers, journal names, research instruments, etc.

Abstracts from nearly half the regularly indexed journals are included. Abstracts are also included for all dissertations, educational software, and audiovisuals.

The CINAHL database is designed with the researcher in mind. The database provides access to methodologies, conceptual frameworks, and data analysis methods used in research studies. The instrumentation field identifies tools used for data collection. The end users may make judgements about the entire study based on the historical reliability or validity of the tool.

Along with regular bibliographic information, the CINAHL database provides additional details of the source such as: author affiliations; producers' names and addresses for software and audiovisuals; the numbers of references and/or recommended readings; a citation index; and selected full text of standards of practice, state nursing journals, nurse practice acts, research instruments, and critical pathways.

Does the database allow you to narrow the search strategy?

In the CINAHL database you can limit the retrieval with more specificity initially, or narrow the search later if too many citations are found.

Topical subheadings, tertiary headings, and check tags can be linked to CINAHL main headings to increase specificity.

Consider specifying document types, journal subsets, update codes, the language, population groupsor gender, or the publication year to narrow your search.

References
1. Corbet, P.K. (1987). Mastering an online database. Medical Reference Services Quarterly 3(1), 4, 6.
2. Quint, B. (1991). Inside a searcher's mind: the stage of an online search, part 1. Online 15(3), 13-18.

Appendix 2

SUBHEADINGS

There are 60 topical subheadings that can be linked to CINAHL subject headings. CINAHL subject headings can be modified by the addition of these subheadings, thereby providing more specific access.

It is Cinahl's policy to assign up to three separate subheadings to a single subject heading. If more than three subheadings are required to cover the content of the article adequately, the subject heading will be assigned without any subheadings. The appropriate subheadings may then be assigned to a minor subject heading.

Not all subheadings can be used with all subject headings; for example, the subheading *prevention and control* is meaningless when linked to the subject heading *Nursing Protocols*. The subcategories of subject headings with which a particular subheading can be combined are identified in parentheses in the subheadings list (below).

In order to avoid incorrect subject heading/subheading combinations, check the CINAHL Subject Heading List scope notes before selecting search terms. Articles will be found under the term *Nursing Costs* but not under *Nursing Care/economics*.

Unless otherwise indicated, subheadings were established prior to 1982.

ABNORMALITIES or AB (83) - Used with organs, regions, and tissues for congenital defects. (A1-10, A14)

ADMINISTRATION or AM - Used for administrative structure and management. Use only for selected headings in the I2 tree. (I2, L, N2-4)

ADMINISTRATION AND DOSAGE or AD - Used with drugs and selected plant products for dosage forms, routes of administration, frequency and duration of administration, quantity of medication, and the effects of these factors. (B6, D)

ADVERSE EFFECTS or AE - Used with drugs, chemicals, plants, and manufactured products for undesirable reactions occurring in normal usage or accepted dosage. Also used for adverse effects or complications of diagnostic, therapeutic, anesthetic, surgical, or other procedures. Excludes contraindications for which "contraindications" is used. Excludes poisoning for which "poisoning" is used. (B6, D, E, F4, G3, H, I3, J)

ANALOGS AND DERIVATIVES or AA (92) - Used with drugs and chemicals for substances that share the same parent molecule or have similar electronic structures but differ by the addition or substitution of other atoms or molecules. It is used when the specific chemical heading is not available. (D3, D6, D14-18, D20-23)

ANALYSIS or AN - Used for the identification or quantitative determination of a substance or its constituents and the chemical analysis of tissues, tumors, body fluids, organisms, and plants. Includes the analysis of air, water, or other environmental carriers. Includes urinalysis, blood analysis, and cerebrospinal fluid analysis as well as the chemistry or chemical composition of an organ or drug. (A2-16, B1, B3-6, C4, D, G3, J)

ANATOMY AND HISTOLOGY or AH (83) - Used with organs, regions, and tissues for normal descriptive anatomy and histology. (A1-10, A14-16, B2, B6)

ANTAGONISTS AND INHIBITORS or AI (85) - Used with chemicals, drugs, and endogenous substances to indicate substances or agents which counteract their biological effects by any mechanism. (D1-23)

CHEMICALLY INDUCED or CI (83) - Used for diseases, syndromes, abnormalities, or symptoms caused by chemical substances. (C1-20, C23, F3)

CLASSIFICATION or CL (83) - Used for taxonomic or other systematic or hierarchical classification systems. (A11, A15, B-N)

COMPLICATIONS or CO (83) - Used with diseases to indicate conditions that co-exist or follow. (C, F3)

CONTRAINDICATIONS or CT (93) - Used with drugs, chemicals, and biological and physical agents in any disease or physical state that might render their use improper, undesirable, or inadvisable. Used also with contraindicated diagnostic, therapeutic, prophylactic, anesthetic, surgical, or other procedures. (D, E)

DEFICIENCY or DF (98) - Used with endogenous and exogenous substances which are absent or in diminished amount relative to the normal requirement of an organism or a biologic system. Use only for selected headings in the D1 and D11 trees. (D1, D8, D11-12)

DIAGNOSIS or DI - Used for all aspects of diagnosis and assessment, including examination and differential diagnosis. Excludes screening for which "prevention and control" is used, excludes prognosis for which "prognosis" is used. For radiographic diagnosis use "radiography"; for ultrasonic diagnosis use "ultrasonography." (C, F3)

DIAGNOSTIC USE or DU (92) - Used with chemical compounds, drugs, and physical agents for studies of the clinical function of an organ, or for the diagnosis of diseases. (B6, D)

DIET THERAPY or DH (83) - Used with disease headings for dietary or nutritional management. Excludes nutritional support such as enteral feeding and parenteral nutrition, for which "therapy" is used. Excludes use of vitamin or mineral supplements for which "drug therapy" is used. (C, F3)

DRUG EFFECTS or DE (83) - Used with organs, regions, tissues, or organisms and physiological and psychological processes for the effects of drugs. Used with the D tree for endogenous substances only. (A, B1, B3-6, D, F1-2, G4-11)

DRUG THERAPY or DT - Used with disease headings for the treatment of diseases by the administration of drugs or chemicals. (C, F3)

ECONOMICS or EC (83) - Used for the economic aspects of any subject, including all aspects of financial management and fund raising. (C-E, F3-4, G1-3, H-J, L, N2-4)

EDUCATION or ED - Used for educating or teaching about diseases, procedures, services, or programs. Used for education and training in various disciplines and of various classes of people. Use available precoordinated education subject headings for formal educational programs. Use only for selected headings in the I2 tree. (C, E-N)

EMBRYOLOGY or EM (97) - Used with organs, regions, and animal headings for embryologic and fetal development. It is used also with diseases for embryologic factors contributing to postnatal disorders. (A1-10, A14, B2, B6, C)

EPIDEMIOLOGY or EP (91) - Used for the distribution and frequency of diseases, injuries, and other health-related events and their causes in a desired population. Includes incidence, prevalence, endemic, and epidemic outbreaks. Excludes mortality for which "mortality" is used. (C, F1, F3, G3)

EQUIPMENT AND SUPPLIES or ES - Used with diagnostic or therapeutic procedures or specialties/disciplines for the development, utilization, or modification of apparatus, instruments, or equipment. (E1-6, F2, F4, G1-3, H, J, L)

ETHICAL ISSUES or EI (98) - Used with disciplines, procedures, personnel, and other selected headings for ethical aspects. (D-N)

ETHNOLOGY or EH (96) - Used with diseases and selected terms for ethnic, cultural, anthropological, or racial aspects, and with geographic headings to indicate the place of origin of a group of people. (C, F1, F3, Z)

ETIOLOGY or ET (83) - Used with medical and social problems for causation. Includes environmental factors, microorganisms, life style, etc. Also used with nursing diagnoses. (C, F3, G3, I1, P)

EVALUATION or EV - Used with non-disease headings (e.g., behavior mechanisms, physiological processes, programs, disciplines, classes of persons, facilities, and services) for evaluation and assessment. (E, F, G2-12, H-J, L-N, P)

FAMILIAL AND GENETIC or FG (90) - Used for discussion of genetic basis of diseases; diseases occurring in family groups due to environmental factors, including infection and common dietary habits; includes hereditary disease. (C, F1, F3)

HISTORY or HI - Used for the historical aspects of any subject. (B6, C-F, G1-3, H-N)

INJURIES or IN - Used with anatomic headings for wounds and injuries. (A1-10, A14-15)

LEGISLATION AND JURISPRUDENCE or LJ - Used for laws, statutes, ordinances, government regulations, legal issues, and court decisions. (B6, C-F, G1-3, H-J, L-N)

MANPOWER or MA (83) - Used with disciplines and programs for the demand, supply, distribution, recruitment, and use of personnel. (G1-2, I, J, L, N2-4)

METABOLISM or ME (92) - Used with organs, cells, organisms, and diseases for biochemical changes and metabolism. It is also used with drugs and chemicals for catabolic changes. (A2-16, B-D, F3)

METHODS or MT (83) - Used with techniques, procedures, and programs for methods. (E1-6, F2, F4, G1-3, H, J, L, N)

MICROBIOLOGY or MI (97) - Used with organs, animals, and higher plants and with diseases for microbiologic factors or studies. (A, B1-2, B6, C, F3)

MORTALITY or MO (95) - Used with human diseases for mortality statistics. (C, E1-4, F3)

NURSING or NU (84) - Used with diseases and certain physiological processes for nursing care and techniques. Includes nursing care in diagnostic, therapeutic, and preventive procedures. Do not use with "Care" headings in the E2 tree. (C, E, F3, G8)

ORGANIZATIONS or OG (83) - Used with disciplines and classes of persons for associated organizations, societies, agencies, etc. Prefer use with disciplines. (C, E, G2, H, I1-2, K-M, N2)

PATHOLOGY or PA (95) - Used for organ, tissue, or cell structure in disease states. (A1-11, A14-16, C, F3)

PHARMACODYNAMICS or PD (87) - Used with drugs and exogenously administered chemical substances for their actions on tissues and organisms; includes effects upon metabolism, acceleration, or inhibition of biological processes, and the mechanisms of action. (B6, D)

PHYSIOLOGY or PH - Used with organs, tissues, and cells for their normal function. Also used with physical processes and biochemical substances, endogenously produced, for their physiological role. (A, B, D, G4-11, I3)

PHYSIOPATHOLOGY or PP - Used with organs, tissues, cell structures, and disease states for disordered function. (A, C, F3)

POISONING or PO (84) - Used with drugs, chemicals, plants, and industrial materials for human or animal poisoning, acute or chronic, whether the poisoning is accidental, occupational, suicidal, by medication error, or by environmental exposure. (B6, D, J)

PREVENTION AND CONTROL or PC (83) - Used with disease headings for increasing disease resistance, control of transmission agents, prevention and control of environmental hazards, and prevention and control of social factors leading to disease. Includes immunization and screening. (C, F1, F3, G3, I1)

PROGNOSIS or PR (96) - Prospect of survival and recovery from a disease as anticipated from the usual course of that disease or indicated by special features of a particular case. (C, F3)

PSYCHOSOCIAL FACTORS or PF (83) - Used with diseases, psychological processes, techniques, and named groups for psychological, psychiatric, psychosomatic, social, behavioral, and emotional aspects. (C, E1-6, F3, G, I, M, N1-2)

RADIATION EFFECTS or RE (92) - Used for the effects of ionizing and nonionizing radiation upon organisms, organs, tissues, and physiologic processes. It includes the effects of irradiation on drugs and chemicals. (A, B1, B3-6, D, G4-12)

RADIOGRAPHY or RA (83) - Used with organs, regions, and diseases for x-ray examinations.

Includes radionuclide imaging, angiography, and x-ray tomography. Use for radiographic diagnosis. For magnetic resonance imaging use "diagnosis"; for ultrasonic diagnosis use "ultrasonography." (A, C, F3)

RADIOTHERAPY or RT (83) - Used with disease headings for the therapeutic use of ionizing and nonionizing radiation. It includes the use of radioisotope therapy. (C)

REHABILITATION or RH (83) - Used with disease headings and surgical procedures for restoration of function of the individual. (C, E4, F3)

STANDARDS or ST (83) - Used with facilities, personnel, programs, and services for the development, testing, and application of guidelines or standards of adequacy or acceptable performance. Includes standards of practice and health or safety standards in industries or occupations. Used with chemicals or drugs for standards of identification, quality, and potency. (D, E, F4, G-J, L, N)

SURGERY or SU (83) - Used for operative procedures on organs, regions, or tissues for the treatment of diseases, including tissue section by lasers. Excludes transplantation for which "transplantation" is used. (A, C, F3)

SYMPTOMS or SS (96) - Used with diseases and disorders for presenting signs and symptoms or clinical manifestations. (C, F3)

THERAPEUTIC USE or TU (84) - Used with drugs, biological preparations, plants, and physical agents for their use in the prophylaxis and treatment of diseases. (B6, D, H)

THERAPY or TH (83) - Used with diseases for therapies other than specific drug therapy, diet therapy, radiotherapy, rehabilitation, or surgery for which subheadings exist. Also used for materials dealing with multiple therapies. (C, F3)

TRANSMISSION or TM (87) - Used with diseases and microbes for the modes of transmission. (B3-4, C)

TRANSPLANTATION or TR (83) - Used with organs, tissues, or cells for transplantation. (A)

TRENDS or TD (83) - Used for the manner in which a subject changes with time, whether past, present, or future. (C, E, F1, F3-4, G1-3, H-J, L, N)

ULTRASONOGRAPHY or US (92) - Used with organs and regions for ultrasonic imaging and with diseases for ultrasonic diagnosis. Does not include ultrasonic therapy. (A, C, F3)

UTILIZATION or UT (83) - Used with procedures, equipment, programs, facilities, and services for discussions of how and how much they are used. (E, F4, G1-3, H-J, L, N, P)

Appendix 3

TERTIARY HEADINGS

Two other groups of subheadings (also known as tertiary headings) are available – population groups and geographics.

Subject heading/subheading and tertiary heading combination
Like topical subheadings, tertiary headings can be linked directly to CINAHL subject headings. Unlike topical subheadings, however, they can also be linked to the end of a subject heading/subheading combination, e.g.,

POPULATION GROUPS
substance abuse/in adolescence or substance abuse/therapy/in adolescence

GEOGRAPHIC
rehabilitation, nursing/United Kingdom or rehabilitation, nursing/education/United Kingdom

POPULATION GROUP

Use of population group subheadings
A population group subheading is added when the population group is key to the topic under discussion. With some main headings (e.g., *Alzheimer's Disease*), the population group is implicit. In such cases the population group subheading will not be assigned unless the population is other than that which would normally be expected.

POPULATION GROUP SUBHEADINGS

- Fetus – from conception to birth
- Infant, Newborn – birth to 1 month
- Infant – 1-23 months
- Child, Preschool – 2-5 years
- Child – 6-12 years
- Adolescence – 13-18 years
- Adult – 19-44 years
- Middle Age – 45-64 years
- Aged – 65+ years
- Aged – 80 and over
- Male
- Female
- Pregnancy
- Inpatients
- Outpatients

GEOGRAPHIC

The geographic headings (see Z section in the tree structures) are unique in that they are the only index terms assigned either as subheadings or as major or minor headings. If the geographic locations are relevant to the main theme of the article, the geographic term will be assigned as both a subheading and as a minor heading. If the geographic location is incidental, the geographic term will be assigned only as a minor heading. Geographic terms are rarely assigned as major headings.

Appendix 4

DOCUMENT TYPES

As many document types as are appropriate will be assigned to each record. CINAHL document types represent the type of publication being indexed (journal, book, audiovisual, pamphlet, software, dissertation, or research instrument). They can also describe the format of the individual item being indexed (e.g., editorial, research, review) or indicate the presence of some special data (e.g., exam questions, care plan, questionnaire).

Research studies published with one or more commentaries are indexed as a single citation. The appropriate document types (e.g., research, commentary, and response) are assigned by the indexer.

ABSTRACT (92) - indicates material indexed is an abstract. It is used for abstracts of presentations at congresses, conferences, symposia, etc. Use with Bibliography for annotated bibliographies. For materials about abstracting, see CINAHL subject heading: ABSTRACTING AND INDEXING.

ACCREDITATION (97) - indicates document containing information about compliance with accreditation requirements.

ALGORITHM (95) - indicates the presence of an algorithm. For materials about algorithms, see CINAHL subject heading: ALGORITHMS.

ANECDOTE - indicates an informal narrative.

AUDIOVISUAL (93) - indicates an audiovisual. For materials about audiovisuals, see CINAHL subject heading: AUDIOVISUALS.

BIBLIOGRAPHY - indicates the presence of a substantive list of books, audiovisuals, articles, documents, publications, etc., usually on a single topic or related topics. For annotated bibliographies, use with Abstract. For discussions about bibliographies, see CINAHL subject heading: BIBLIOGRAPHY AND REFERENCES.

BIOGRAPHY (85) - indicates a history or an account of the personal and/or professional life of an individual.

BOOK (85) - indicates a book.

BOOK CHAPTER (93) - indicates a chapter, section, or article within a book.

BRIEF ITEM (95) - indicates material of less than one page.

CARE PLAN - indicates the presence of a care plan — i.e., a written plan developed to assure consistent care of an individual patient or for a specific disease. For materials about or how to develop care plans, see CINAHL subject headings: NURSING CARE PLANS or PATIENT CARE PLANS.

CARTOON (95) - indicates a cartoon.

CASE STUDY - indicates a review of a particular condition, disease, or administrative problem. Includes case reports.

CEU (85) - indicates material that has been approved by a professional society for continuing education credit. May be dated or non-dated. CEU material will be double indexed under the CINAHL subject heading EDUCATION, CONTINUING (CREDIT) as well as under the appropriate subject terms.

CLASSIFICATION TERM (98) - indicates the presence of a NANDA Nursing Diagnosis, IOWA Nursing Intervention or SABA Home Health Care Nursing Diagnosis or Intervention classification term and scope note, together with a CINAHL editorial search suggestion.

CLINICAL INNOVATIONS (97) - indicates document which describes new approaches to patient care.

CLINICAL TRIAL (98) - indicates the research study is a clinical trial, a randomized clinical trial, or a randomized controlled trial. Coordinate with the document type Research.

CODE OF ETHICS (98) - indicates material indexed is a professional code of ethics, or indicates the presence of a professional code of ethics or conduct. For discussions about professional codes of ethics or conduct, see CINAHL subject headings ETHICS; ETHICS, MEDICAL; or ETHICS, NURSING.

COMMENTARY - indicates a commentary – i.e., a comment on another written article.

COMPUTER PROGRAM (86) - indicates the presence of a written computer program. For materials about computer programs, see CINAHL subject heading: SOFTWARE or specifics.

CONSUMER/PATIENT TEACHING MATERIALS (97) - indicates the presence of various teaching/educational/learning materials for the consumer or patient. Use Teaching Materials for materials used for student education or staff development. For discussions about consumer/patient teaching materials, see CINAHL subject headings: TEACHING MATERIALS and PATIENT EDUCATION.

CORRECTED ARTICLE (93) - indicates an article that has been republished in order to correct, amplify, or restore text and data from the originally published article.

CRITICAL PATH (95) - indicates material indexed is a critical path or care map, or indicates the presence of a critical path or care map. For discussions about critical paths or care maps, see CINAHL subject heading: CRITICAL PATH.

DIAGNOSTIC IMAGES (97) - indicates the presence of images produced by radiography, magnetic resonance imaging, ultrasonography, or other diagnostic imaging procedures.

DIRECTORIES (96) - indicates names and addresses of various persons, agencies, schools, and other institutions. For discussions about directories, see CINAHL subject heading: INFORMATION RESOURCES.

DOCTORAL DISSERTATION (90) - indicates a doctoral dissertation or thesis. For discussions about dissertations, see CINAHL subject heading: THESES AND DISSERTATIONS.

DRUGS (98) - indicates the presence of a description of a drug; includes nursing and other healthcare personnel considerations and patient information.

EDITORIAL - indicates an editorial. Includes guest editorials and presidents' messages.

EQUATIONS & FORMULAS (97) - indicates the presence of mathematical equations or formulas.

EXAM QUESTIONS - indicates the presence of sample exams or CEU questions.

FORMS - indicates the presence of sample forms. For materials about forms, see CINAHL subject heading: DOCUMENTATION or specifics.

GAMES (97) - indicates the presence of a word search, crossword puzzle, maze, or other type of game. For discussions about games, see CINAHL subject heading: GAMES AND SIMULATIONS.

GLOSSARY (96) - indicates lists of words with definitions.

HISTORICAL MATERIAL (92) - indicates material (or a portion thereof) that has been reprinted from an earlier work of historical interest.

INTERVIEW (85) - indicates an interview.

JOURNAL ARTICLE - indicates material published in a journal. For discussions about journals, see CINAHL subject heading: SERIAL PUBLICATIONS.

JOURNAL DESCRIPTION (98) - indicates the presence of a description of a journal title, including the scope and audience of the journal.

LEGAL CASES (97) - indicates the inclusion of a court case or court cases.

LETTER (91) - indicates letters to the editor that are substantive in nature.

MASTERS THESIS (98) - indicates a master's thesis or dissertation.

NURSE PRACTICE ACTS (96) - indicates material indexed is a nurse practice act or indicates the presence of a nurse practice act within the material. Use Practice Acts for other than nurse practice acts. For discussions about nurse practice acts, see CINAHL subject heading: NURSE PRACTICE ACTS.

NURSING DIAGNOSES (88) - indicates material that contains nursing diagnoses as a substantive part of a care plan, case study, or in relation to the subject being discussed. For materials about nursing diagnosis, see CINAHL subject heading: NURSING DIAGNOSIS or specifics.

NURSING INTERVENTIONS (94) - indicates material that contains nursing interventions as a substantive part of a care plan, case study, or in relation to the subject being discussed. For materials about nursing interventions, see CINAHL subject heading: NURSING INTERVENTIONS or specifics.

OBITUARY (85) - indicates an obituary.

OTHER (94) - indicates miscellaneous material not yet categorized.

OVERALL (95) - indicates material being indexed contains multiple articles or chapters on the same topic.

PAMPHLET (85) - indicates a pamphlet.

PAMPHLET CHAPTER (93) - indicates a chapter, section, or article within a pamphlet.

PICTORIAL - indicates the presence of substantive photographs, pictures, or medical illustrations.

POETRY (96) - indicates a poem or poems.

PRACTICE ACTS (97) - indicates material indexed is a practice act or indicates the presence of a practice act within the material. Use Nurse Practice Acts for nurse practice acts.

PRACTICE GUIDELINES (97) - indicates the presence of practice guidelines. For materials about practice guidelines, see CINAHL subject heading: PRACTICE GUIDELINES.

PROCEEDINGS (92) - indicates collection of papers presented at conferences, symposia, congresses, meetings, etc. Such papers may be published in full or in an edited or revised form. Also includes collection of abstracts of papers presented at such conferences, etc.

PROTOCOL (84) - indicates the presence of a protocol – i.e., written plans specifying the methods to be followed in performing various procedures or in conducting research. For materials about protocols, see CINAHL subject headings: PROTOCOLS, NURSING PROTOCOLS, or RESEARCH PROTOCOLS.

QUESTIONNAIRE - indicates the presence of a sample questionnaire. For materials about questionnaires, see CINAHL subject heading: QUESTIONNAIRES.

RESEARCH - indicates a research study containing data collection, methodology, discussion of results, etc. For materials about or how to conduct a research study, see specific CINAHL subject headings, such as CLINICAL NURSING RESEARCH or RESEARCH, MEDICAL.

RESEARCH INSTRUMENT (95) - indicates material indexed is a research instrument. To indicate the use of instruments in a body of work, search electronically using the particular name. For material about research instruments, see CINAHL subject heading: RESEARCH INSTRUMENTS or specifics.

RESPONSE - indicates material written in response to a commentary.

REVIEW (88) - indicates a substantial review of the literature.

SOFTWARE (92) - indicates a piece of educational software [listed in electronic versions only]. For materials about software, see CINAHL subject heading: SOFTWARE or specifics.

STANDARDS (92) - indicates a formal standard of practice or position paper issued by a professional organization. For materials discussing practice standards, see CINAHL subheading "/standards" with appropriate subject heading(s).

STATISTICS - indicates the presence of substantive statistical data applicable outside the context of a research study. For materials about statistics, see CINAHL subject heading: STATISTICS.

SYSTEMATIC REVIEW (98) - indicates a research process in which a concept is identified and the research which has studied it is analyzed and evaluated. The results of this research are synthesized to present the current state of knowledge regarding the concept. Includes integrated or integrative reviews. If the material is a research study, coordinate with document type Research. For materials about Systematic Reviews, see CINAHL subject heading SYSTEMATIC REVIEW.

TABLES/CHARTS (85) - indicates the presence of tables and/or charts.

TEACHING MATERIALS - indicates the presence of various teaching/educational/learning materials for students, health personnel, or individuals in various other disciplines. Use Consumer/Patient Teaching Materials for materials used to educate the consumer or patient. For discussions about teaching materials, see CINAHL subject headings: TEACHING MATERIALS or TEACHING MATERIALS, CLINICAL.

TRACINGS (95) - indicates a graphic record produced by an instrument capable of making a visual record of movement. Included here are ECG, EEG, EMG tracings, and waveforms.

WEBSITE (98) - indicates material indexed is a description of a website(s), or indicates a list of websites on a single topic or related topics.

Appendix 5

OTHER ACCESS POINTS WITHIN THE CINAHL® DATABASE

Subject Focus Fields

Search by the series titles
Series titles for books, pamphlets, and journals are available and are keyword searchable.

Search for new topics that have not been assigned subject headings
The terms in process field includes vocabulary terms (only main headings, no subheadings) that are being considered for inclusion in next year's subject heading list.

Bibliographic Fields

Search for contributors, corporate authors, or government agency authors
Multi-authored books indexed at chapter level list the author(s) of the specific chapter including the name of the first editor. If there is more than one editor the words "et al" will be added. Books not indexed at the chapter level will list the name(s) of the editor(s), but not the contributors.

Corporate names are entered as they appear in the article. Subordinate bodies (including government agencies) are entered as subheadings of the name of the bodies to which they are subordinate when:

- The name contains more than one term that implies that it is part of another, e.g., Department, Division, Section, Branch, Agency, etc.
- The name indicates a geographic, chronological, numbered, or lettered subdivision, e.g., Region 5, etc.
- The name does not contain the name of the government.
- The name does not convey the name of the corporate body.
- The name includes the entire name of the higher or related term, e.g., Yale University Library.

The bodies listed above are entered as a subheading of the lowest element in the hierarchy, e.g.,

US Department of Health & Human Services. Public Health Services. Agency for Health Care Policy & Research Services will be entered as: US Public Health Services. Agency For Health Care Policy Research.

Search to see how often an author or article has been cited in the literature
The author(s), title, and source for references, cited at the end of articles in selected nursing and allied health journals, are included in the CINAHL® database.

Search for an accession number
Cinahl assigns a unique ten-digit number to each record in the database. These numbers can be used by you to locate specific records.

Search for a topic in a specific journal
The source field for journal records includes the full journal title and/or journal title abbreviation, publication year, volume and issue number, pagination, and references. This information is essential for locating the journal article in the library.

Fields with Additional Information

Search for a particular hospital or university (author affiliation field) doing research of interest to you
The business address is entered for the first author of a journal article, pamphlet, book, or book chapter.

Search for an answer to a specific question or to ascertain what is included in an overall record
To provide comprehensive coverage of selected regular columns in nursing and allied health journals, a table of contents field has been provided electronically. The author (if any), title of the item, and pagination are provided. Items in regular columns cover product information, new drugs, nursing practice issues, etc.

Search for research instruments or clinical assessment tools used in research studies
Search the instrumentation field to locate research studies which use specific research instruments.

Search for funding information
Funding information can be found in the grant information field. When there is a grant or partial grant indicated the subject heading *Funding Source* will always be used as a minor subject heading.

Search for websites, legal cases, and reviews of journal articles
You can find information on specific websites or legal cases, or locate book and journal reviews by searching the specific fields (see Notes on Records on pages 36-39).

NOTES

CD-ROM QUICK START

Enclosed is an instructional CD-ROM that will explain the Thesaurus as referred to on page 20.

To play this CD-ROM, you will need a computer that has the following:

1. DOS 5.0 or above *or* Windows 3.1 or later *or* Macintosh System 7.0 or later
2. A QuickTime movie viewer*
3. 16-bit sound card and speakers
4. 2x CD-ROM drive or faster
5. If QuickTime is to be installed, Windows 3.x: 5 megabytes free hard drive space; Windows 95: 15 megabytes free hard drive space

If you do not have a QuickTime movie viewer and you are using a PC, two have been bundled for your convenience. Qteasy16.exe for Windows 3.x and Qt32.exe for Windows 95/98/NT are located on the CD-ROM.

INSTALLING QUICKTIME

Windows 3.x

1. After placing the Cinahl CD into your CD-ROM drive, open File Manager (usually located in the Main program group)
2. Click on the CD-ROM drive that contains the Cinahl CD
3. Double-click on the Qtease16.exe installation file
4. Follow the on-screen instructions for installing QuickTime onto your computer

Windows 95/98/NT

1. After placing the Cinahl CD into your CD-ROM drive, double click on My Computer (located on your desktop)
2. Double click on the CD-ROM drive labeled Cinahl_CD
3. Double click on the Qt32.exe installation file
4. Follow the on-screen instructions for installing QuickTime onto your computer

WATCHING THE VIDEO

This video is best viewed at 640x480 resolution and 256 colors. Consult your video card's documentation on how to change video resolutions and color depth.

Windows 3.x

1. With the SEE THE CITES WITH CINAHL CD in your CD-ROM drive, open File Manager (usually located in your Main program group)
2. Click on the CD-ROM drive that contains the SEE THE CITES WITH CINAHL CD. Double-click on the Cinahl.mov file and enjoy the show

Windows 95

1. With the SEE THE CITES WITH CINAHL CD in your CD-ROM drive, double-click on My Computer (on your desktop)
2. Double-click on the CD-ROM drive labeled Cinahl_CD
3. Double-click on the Cinahl.mov file and enjoy the show

Macintosh

1. Insert the SEE THE CITES WITH CINAHL CD into your CD-ROM drive
2. Double-click on the Cinahl CD icon that appears on your desktop
3. Double-click on the Cinahl.mov file and enjoy the show